TABLE OF CONTENTS

18. Short-term gratification = long-term frustration

19. Time = money

20. Break the rules and beat the fools

21. Eating nuts? Are you completely nuts?!

22. Just do it! Sounds great, but do what, Alex?

23. Snoozing means losing

24. Life is all about the small things

25. I want to hug everybody who has ever hurt me

26. Don't get bitter! Get better!

27. There's only one opponent that I need to beat. I'm looking at him in the mirror.

28. Humanity is the only species on this entire planet with self- destructive behavior

29. . You're not tired, you're just uninspired

30. You can read 500 blogs and still achieve nothing

31. I don't go with the flow. I flow with the go.

32. Reality shows are just a way to escape from your own problems

33. My way is a way, not *the* way

34. (Never) say thank you to the people who've hurt you

35. Be ego-less with an ego

36. Eat your loss, come back like a boss

37. You can see but be blind. You can hear but be deaf. You can be alive yet completely dead.

38. Stop looking and you'll find what you've been

looking for all along

39.   Positive emotions are just as dangerous as negative ones

40.   You have free will, but your fate is determined

41.   There's only one way to leave a legacy

42.   People who don't better themselves become parents from books on the shelves.

43.   You'll always be a product of your environment, so make sure that you're a quality product

44.   The show must go on

45.   It's perfectly OK to be imperfect

46.   Your mind is a tool. It can be used for self-destruction.

47.   A lot of guys like clingy girls until they get cheated on

48.   Progress equals life, stagnation equals death

49.   Be selfish in a good way. It's safe to say that life is better that way.

50.   Sometimes you have to spend time on yourself to realize how happy and blessed you really are

51.   The feeling of frustration is an opportunity to change. Use it wisely.

52.   Wasting energy on negative thoughts will completely exhaust you

53.   Purpose gives meaning to life

54.   Not living in line with your purpose will make you sick

55.   People who're unhappily single mainly don't

know how to use their time wisely

56.   Follow your gut and you won't get stuck in a rut

57.   Suffering is a choice

58.   Corny quotes are really corny, but they can be 100% true

59.   My stumbling stone is my stepping stone, too

60.   Learn to value your time or somebody else will teach you

61.   Mo' money, mo' problems. Mo' time, mo' money.

62.   You don't need permission. Go fucking get it!

63.   The way you view the world say a lot about you

64.   The garden analogy, life & the world

65.   The best piece of advice for your younger self

66.   Live in the now. Learn from the past. Think about the future.

67.   The best time to start is right now and the second best time is right now, too

68.   Second guessing yourself is not an option

69.   One thing or nothing at all?

70.   Enjoy the process

71.   Helping people is the best thing there is

72.   Your mind controls your body, not the other way around

73.   Bored? How can you be bored in this day and age?

74.   Do what you like and forget about the money

75.   The subtle art of not giving a flying fuck

76.   My biggest fear turns out to be my biggest motivation

77.   Every innovator will attract more than one hater

78.   Misery loves some company in a company

79.   Find an environment that challenges you

80.   Tactical unemployment, a.k.a. "the sabbatical year."

81.   You can't defeat me, so why even bother?

82.   People put on an act despite never receive being eligible to win an Oscar

83.   The nice guy will always finish last because nice guys are assholes

84.   There's a place where the frustrated people gather. It's called "the comment section."

85.   . You have two lives, but most people only live one

86.   Being a loser takes zero effort, but it's a hard life

87.   Contradicting yourself is not as bad as you might think

88.   Are you really unworldly or just smarter than the others?

89.   You might like to twerk, but I love hard work

90.   Learn to sweat. The more you sweat, the luckier you get.

91.   Passion will get you nowhere in life

92.   Only a fool will chase everything that's cool

93.   Famous for nothing to get shit for free

94.   Listen to comprehend instead of with the intent to reply

95.   *The Ex-Files*: are you completely doomed?

96.   Be the writer of your own story

97.   So, tell me why are you waiting on the perfect Monday?

98.   Just ask. Be proactive!

99.   Did someone disappoint you or did you do it to yourself?

100.   The most powerful supplement on earth

101.   Learn to be alone

102.   *AYW*: Access Your "Why"

103.   The only way to avoid haters

104.   Haters make you famous

105.   Some people want to see you go down

106.   Mindset hack to get you back on track

107.   Don't talk, just walk

108.   Male feminists are the worst

109.   Hey, Alex, are you part of (insert any kind of popular movement)?

110.   The power of acceptance

111.   Dumb and dumber

112.   Pick the right wife for the sake of your life

113.   Read books and forget about the looks

114.   Why do most people have drunk personalities?

115.   People are always looking for the next big thing and they never find it

139. I will never play the lottery.

140. Family is a fancy word

141. You're wired to be tired

142. I learned some valuable lessons after a series of injuries

143. Do it now instead of tomorrow and you won't feel sorrow

144. Forgiveness is a very powerful tool

145. Respect is an extremely thoughtful act

146. Choices shape your life whether you like it or not

147. A fancy degree will never impress me

148. Look at results, not at ranks

149. The process is a lot more addictive than the end result

150. The generation that rejects relations lives in frustration

151. Mental health is crucial in life

152. Karma will catch up with you (and you deserve it)

153. A win or a loss in life shouldn't define who you are

154. How to handle a loss like a boss

155. Being on a win streak is dangerous

156. Forgot about a win or a loss

157. Traveling is the most subtle form of escapism

158. Leading an unhappy life with a non- future wife

159. Dream killers are egocentric people without realizing it

160. There's something wrong with the education system

161. Losers focus on winners, winners focus on winning

162. Small talk is boring

163. Excuses will make sure that you'll never grow

164. My way is a way, but it's not the way (part II)

165. Always be extremely grateful

166. Perception defines your reality

167. Pride serves the ego, but it doesn't serve you

168. You don't see skin color? Are you fucking blind??

169. The craving for comfort is a threat to society

170. The craving for comfort and getting into shape

171. Work your ass off in everything you do

172. Are you dead or alive? The answer might shock you!

173. You can't outrun fear, but can you conquer it?

174. A story about a bike ride

175. The bike analogy that'll change your life forever

176. I've never lost a street fight. Here's how I do it:

177. Never go three days without exercise

178. Fail forward instead of falling forward

179. It all starts with one. "One what, Alex?"

180. What is the meaning of a day?

point

270. Most people love and hate the weekend at the same time

271. Cheers to the fucking weekend

272. Unhappiness can make you do great things

273. What doesn't kill you makes you stronger

274. Stuck in a rut? Follow your gut!

275. Where most people fail is before they even start

276. Follow your gut or keep your mouth shut

277. Save your drama for your mama

278. So tell me again: why are you waiting on the perfect Monday?

279. Do you really want it? I don't think so.

280. Balance is the key to a happy life

281. Life & the quest to find balance

282. It's good, it's bad, it's a little bit of both

283. Balance & learning

284. The reason why you're facing regret

285. Take the bet and beat regret

286. The magic of words

287. The magic of words? Feed the hollow ones to the birds.

288. Call people out on their bullshit

289. The magic of thoughts

290. Take the bet, pick a goal to set

291. Being cheap is a very expensive lifestyle

292. You'll start to fade if you're not mentally

challenged

293.　People keep telling me that I've changed. I tell them that they're still the same.

294.　You'll face haters when you take action. You'll face regret when you don't take action. Pick your poison.

295.　Most people will do anything to get in shape

296.　Age is either a number or an excuse

297.　People always find an excuse to judge others but never to better themselves

298.　Go your own way because the right people will stay and the wrong people will go away

299.　Action is the highway to confidence. Waiting is the highway to self-doubt.

300.　Single and assuming to be ready to mingle

301.　I live in the now, learn from the past and work for the future

302.　Politicians are high-paid clowns who wear expensives suit instead red noses

303.　Revenge hurts the other person once while it hurts you twice

304.　People claim that the sky is the limit, but we've been on the moon

305.　People who hate their mornings hate their lives

306.　The truth hurts you in the short term while lies hurt you in the long term. Pick your poison.

307.　You are what you repeatedly do, so don't do useless stuff

308. "No" means no and "yes" means yes

309. Never bite a helping hand

310. Be open-minded and close-minded at the same time

311. Only people who read between the lines will be completely fine

312. Your mind is like a parachute. You're in trouble when it's not open.

313. You can't pour more water in a cup that's already full

314. Every great story starts with failure or adversity not with vodka

315. You're a product of your actions, not your feelings

316. "Dream, believe, achieve" doesn't work

317. The problem is that you assume you've got time while time it's actually running out

318. You can be wealthy yet completely poor. You can be poor yet extremely wealthy.

319. Progress beats pain

320. Find your "why" and the "how" will take care of itself

321. People would rather google an excuse than actually put in the work

322. Cheap shots from a cheap guy

323. Writing this book was not that hard

324. Instant gratification leads to long-term frustration

344.   Friends? Everybody is replaceable.

345.   Hard work pays off in the long run

346.   353. Do what you love to get rid of fear

347.   354. There's always a solution but never a problem

348.   Slow progress is progress

349.   You need a purpose to be happy in life

350.   Do you work to live or live to work?

351.   Everything I do won't be for you.

352.   Are you feeling sad and lonely on Valentine's Day?

353.   Pain is cruel, but you can use it as fuel.

354.   So tell me, do you count on faith to solve things?

355.   How can you live if you never challenge your beliefs?

356.   Why I actually dislike the term "alpha male"

357.   Honesty is a very expensive gift.

358.   Write, because it heals the soul and relaxes the mind.

359.   Why you should call people out on their bullshit

360.   The word "adult" means absolutely nothing

361.   Most adults are arrogant and question nothing

362.   Most adults envy other adults for their "stuff"

363.   Most adults can't handle their own lives or liquor

364.   Most adults avoid responsibilities like the plague

◆ ◆ ◆

1. INTRODUCTION

It's been a long time since my first book was released, but during that time I was lucky enough to pick up a lot more followers on social media. The one topic that usually gets brought up by these new followers is that some just didn't really "get" my quotes. So I decided to repackage all 366 quotes and bundle them all together with the right explanation. In that way, you'll have a better chance to implement what's to be learned from these mini-lessons into your own life. You'll quickly notice that there's always a hidden meaning behind these quotes and that they're not as opaque as you might assume. My suggestion for this book is that you process one quote a day until you hit the end of the year. It might be too much if you read the book all at once, but you're free to do as you please. Whatever you do, give consideration to how each of these ideas plays a part in your own life.

Enjoy,

Alex (www.zerotoalpha.com)

2. VANITY LEADS TO INSANITY

I wrote this after Instagram really started to boom. Tons of people were doing everything they could to get more and more likes, leading to extreme vanity. These people basically aim to be perfect all the time and have completely lost their sense of reality. I mean, we all have imperfect lives, right? But what famous Instagrammer wants to admit to his millions of followers that it's OK to be anything but flawless?

There's nothing wrong with trying to build an audience on Instagram or on any other social media. It's a way to make a living, but beware of your ego becoming bound to this. Make a clear distinction between the real and virtual worlds. Make sure that your reality doesn't turn into a virtual reality. It's OK to fail. It's OK to have a bad hair day. It's OK to get your ass kicked in sparring. Severe depression is right around the corner if you try to live like this.

3. WHEN YOU COMPLAIN, YOU ACCEPT UNNECESSARY PAIN

This is a quote from one of my earliest blogposts and, in my opinion, is a vital truth.

We will all face a point in our lives in which we hit rock bottom. But rock bottom should be your starting point, not where you finish. So many people get caught up in their own complaints that they never change anything about the situation. Many will complain to others who comfort them and tell them that they're right. They're essentially looking for a person to tell them that life is unfair and that they were born cursed with unluckiness. This is a classic self-fulfilling prophecy.

Catch yourself or others next time there's an urge to complain. You're only hurting yourself more and more by complaining. It's braver to accept it, learn the lesson and move on.

A wise man once said, "sometimes you just need to keep standing." He was absolutely right. Complaining never solved a single problem, so why are you even doing it?

4. WHEN YOU WHINE, YOU SHOW A LACK OF SPINE

I picked up a lot of life lessons from my grandfather and other great mentors. There's one common thread through all their wisdom: they each agree that nobody likes men without a spine.

People who whine keep on complaining over and over again about the same problem. It's next-level complaining and also proves the weakness of our generation. The major problem with this approach is that you completely repel those who could actually help you.

Why? Because nobody likes a whiner. Nobody likes a person who's whining a whole year about the same problem. You're going to have a hard time in life if you don't get this. Life tends to push people around who whine a lot until they break or stand up and do something about it. So why are you still whining?

5. SHOULDN'T YOU DO BARBELL CURLS INSTEAD OF CHASING GIRLS?

I took this one from my most popular blog post so far. Many of my readers assumed that I was pushing people into fitness to make sure that they would be more popular. This wasn't the case.

I was actually trying to communicate that you should aim to better yourself before you date again. Girls can never be your number-one priority. You can't be successful in life and chase girls at the same time. You might think that it's cool to get a one-night stand every single weekend, but how long can you live your life like this? Is it getting you closer to a goal? Are you feeling satisfied or left wanting something more after all these experiences?

This might be a lot to process, but you should focus on yourself and your projects. Be selfish in a good way. The right woman will come in due time and it'll save you a ton of frustrating dates. That's what we call a win-win, right?

6. I SLEEP WHEN I'M TIRED, NOT WHEN IT'S TIME

Many people don't have a sleep schedule at all, so this one could be tricky to relate to for them.

Most of the time, I sleep eight hours a night, but I usually feel a little tired at noon or soon after noon. So, I take a 10-minute nap when I feel this way. I could just down a coffee or an energy drink, but this is the wrong way to go. You should rest when you're tired.

I'm pretty sure that this will pay off in the long run. A lot of athletes do it, so why aren't you? Because it isn't cool? Well, being healthy will never be cool. It isn't Instagrammable, but it'll leave you feeling great. Why not give it a shot? Take a nap and feel completely energized afterwards. Don't forget to eat something after the nap, otherwise you'll feel drowsy.

7. I EAT WHEN I'M HUNGRY AND DRINK WHEN I'M THIRSTY

People laughed when I shared this quote because it's common sense, right? Well, this habit might not be as common as you might think.

Many of us eat when we should eat, according to the clock. Or we eat every three hours while counting calories and drinking *x* amount of water.

I don't do any of that. I eat when I'm really hungry and drink when I'm really thirsty. I do this until I'm completely satisfied and good to go.

So no, I don't count calories and I don't track my water intake. My main takeaway from the experience of these habits? We need to listen to our bodies; they're always telling us something.

8. COMFORT KILLS (BUT IT ALSO PAYS THE BILLS)

There's no growth when you're constantly pursuing comfort. I mean, just look at the things that make you comfortable. All these things require zero effort from you. You just consume their comfort and live your convenient life.

It's easy to fall into this lifestyle. We want to follow the herd. We expect to go to college and end up doing a job that we don't like doing.

The problem is that this same job actually makes sure that you get by pretty easily as well. It ensures that you're able to pay the bills and buy some food. That's the problem that most people don't seem to get. It's hard to change your life when you're comfortable. It's hard to force yourself to get up early when you wake up in a warm bed. What should we change? Start with your attitude towards comfort. Comfort is not your friend.

9. DON'T ACT LIKE A BLACK BELT WHEN YOU CAN'T EVEN TIE A WHITE ONE

Some people want to portray themselves as experts while they actually know next to nothing about the subject matter. This is something really weird that seems to happen with some people. It's a really strange tendency that makes us act this way.

Some people act like a doctor, dietician and political leader in the same day. They all act like they know so much. But in reality, they're in bad shape, they have bad health, and they don't really understand reality.

Never give advice on things that you've never done yourself. Never tell people how they should do something while they've been doing it effectively their entire lives. I'm not going to tell Floyd Mayweather how to box or Rickson Gracie how to grapple. I would sit down and listen to them because they're full of knowledge. Look to learn new things instead of impressing others.

10. LONELINESS IS A PAINFUL BOOMERANG

There's a saying that goes like this: "you're in bad company if you're feeling lonely."

This is actually true. A lot of people do everything they can to escape this feeling, but they mostly just end up even worse off. Just look at all the lonely people who try to drink this feeling away. They assume that they're fine while they're drunk, but eventually this feeling catches up with them over time and smacks them right in the face.

The main truth to know here is that you shouldn't try to escape your problems, and especially not with alcohol or drugs. You'll slowly kill yourself overtime. The cure for the pain is always within the pain.

11. THE CURE FOR THE PAIN IS IN THE PAIN

Let's face it: nobody likes to be hurt.

And still, it happens to all of us, multiple times throughout a lifetime. I mean, who didn't feel heartbroken after they got dumped for the first time? I still remember the first time that my heart got crushed. I got dumped, then she came back months later and cheated on me. It was a devastating experience and I did everything to escape the pain.

The trouble was that the trust problems were left unresolved. And guess what? She returned one year later and did the same thing to me again. Now I was crushed and ashamed of myself. I hadn't made any progress in a whole year.

Some time after that, I burned out and developed suicidal tendencies. Everything changed the moment that I accepted and acknowledged my pain. I had been carrying extra weight for a whole year and I didn't even realize it. You can run all you want, but the obstacle will remain. I just learned that through the obstacle was the way.

12. YOU CAN SAY SORRY AS MUCH AS YOU WANT, BUT IT WON'T MATTER

Sometimes people put on shitty behavior and get away with it because they just say "sorry" without even meaning the sentiment. To those people, I say why don't you feed your hollow words to the birds.

When I judge others, I don't analyze their words. I take a look at their actions and don't give a damn about the rest. You can never hide your true intentions if you're forced to take action. Some people might get away with shitty behavior with me once, but I'll never let them get away with it twice. I always kick them out of my life after they treat me wrongly for the second time.

Some people think this is harsh, but it's actually a way of making sure that you don't have unwanted drama in your life. Some people will never change, so you'd better kick them out if they treat you badly.

13. FIGHTING AND LIFE HAVE A LOT IN COMMON

I compare everything to fighting, but most others don't see the resemblance between combat and life. A lot of people don't want to do combat sports for one simple reason: they want to hit and not get hit.

This is a wrong mindset if you ask me. Getting hit is a part of the game, but you can minimize the impact or damage that you take in. You can never avoid getting hit, just as you can never avoid adversity and failure.

That's why I compare fighting to life all the time. People want to punch all the time or, in other words, they always want "the good." But they never want to get hit or face "the bad." It's going to happen anyways, so why don't you just bite down on your mouthpiece and start fighting back? You need to stand up and fight back, otherwise life will knock you out stone-cold.

14. SWING IT IF YOU CAN'T WING IT!

I wrote this after a horrible sparring session. I realized that I would have been ahead on the scorecards if this were to have been an actual fight. I wasn't as creative as I usually am, and I knew that creativity wasn't going to magically appear anytime soon.

Basically, I realized that I couldn't wing it, I was gonna have to swing for it. This means that I had to just bite down on my mouthpiece and make it as dirty as possible just to show what I was made of if nothing else.

This is a mindset that also carries over in life. Sometimes you need to keep on pushing no matter what. You need to realize that you can never give up, even if you're already on your knees. The main thing that I learned during that sparring session was that I am able to push on when times get really tough. It's an important lesson for every person to learn.

15. I START MY DAY FIGHTING

People always assume that I'm talking about shadow-boxing in this quote, but I'm not.

Everybody starts the day with a fight. Getting up is literally the first fight of the day. You're in a warm, comfortable bed and you need to convince yourself that you should get up and get hustling. The only problem is that you need to do this 365 days a year and it never become easy.

Be aware of this next time you're eager to stay in bed. There's no need to stay in bed if you're not sick. Start your day fighting and you will be ready for anything that comes your way.

16. YOU ARE JUST AS STRONG AS THE ACTIONS YOU TAKE

Mike Tyson was a beast in the ring but always lost when he was really tested (five times, in fact). This comes from legendary boxing trainer and Tyson's former trainer, Teddy Atlas.

And it's true! He could do cocaine all weekend and beat up weaker people, but those actions didn't make him stronger. The problem with all these weak actions is that they turn you into a weak person. So guess what happens when you get tested? That's right, you'll do what every weak person would do. You'll look for the easy way out.

Always take the high road in life. Always do the right thing no matter how hard it may be. This will turn you into a stronger person and make sure that you always find the right solution when you're facing hard times.

17. I'M GLAD THAT I DON'T HAVE RICH PARENTS. THEY'RE A CURSE.

People always want what they don't have. They always want extremely wealthy parents because they think that money will solve every single problem. Newsflash: it won't solve a single problem (and it might even kill your happiness as a consequence).

A lot of rich kids are doing drugs because they're extremely unhappy. I mean, who could be happy if their source of happiness is linked to "stuff"? Rich kids are constantly somewhere between the state of momentary happiness and complete emptiness.

So be careful what you wish for, because you might not get what you actually want.

18. SHORT-TERM GRATIFICATION = LONG-TERM FRUSTRATION

People so often fail to think long-term when they take certain actions. So they do whatever gives them pleasure in that particular moment and regret it afterwards.

You always have a choice when you take a certain action, so try to think how it'll affect you in the long run. Will binging Netflix shows for the fifth night in a row make you feel better? I highly doubt it! But the workout that you've been putting off for the last five days will.

Sometimes you've just got to realize that the best things in life aren't always the most fun ones to start with. I don't always feel like training, but I do it anyways because I always feel happy afterwards. I wouldn't have the same feeling if I binged a whole season of *Friends*. Trade short-term gratifications for long-term ones.

19. TIME = MONEY

This is so misunderstood! A lot of people have even bashed this quote because it's so often used by managers and people who're running a business. Most people assume that the emphasis of this quote is on the money part, but it isn't.

The focal point is time, because time is your most valuable asset.

There's enough money in the world to make everybody a millionaire. You can even regain lost money, but how about time? How much time have you actually regained? None of it, right?

When I work overtime and have to choose between more overtime (money) or time off, I take time off because I value my time more than I value money. I can do a lot more useful stuff in that time, which can even lead to extra income. Most people don't get this, so that's why they take the paycheck.

20. BREAK THE RULES AND BEAT THE FOOLS

We've been corrupted by the school system and we don't even realize it.

School teaches us to follow the rules and, in the process, kills all creativity. People who do this are textbook people who follow the textbook way. Listen, there is nothing wrong with the textbook way because it has proven to work over and over again. But it's predictable as well.

The textbook way is not how I approach MMA. I mostly spar with my hands down and do unorthodox stuff. You can't prepare for the things that you can't predict and that's why it works. My old trainer always told me that my style would never work, while my new trainer just fine-tuned it.

Guess what happened after I changed camps? I progressed a lot faster because I had a lot more freedom to be creative.

Some people might do well with textbook trainers, but I need freedom to express myself. That's probably why I sucked in school.

21. EATING NUTS? ARE YOU COMPLETELY NUTS?!

This was a diss I wrote to some blogger who claimed that you shouldn't eat nuts because it was supposed to lower your testosterone levels.

Those guys were taking it to the extreme, but there's also a lesson here: never take things to the extreme. Some nuts might lower your testosterone, and some foods might be unhealthy, but you won't die if you eat them once in a while. I eat unhealthy foods from time to time; hell, I even eat some nuts, too.

Don't listen to people who're too much on the extreme. They'll mostly never live pleasant lives (and they usually don't even realize it).

22. JUST DO IT! SOUNDS GREAT, BUT DO WHAT, ALEX?

People tend to ask others for advice all the time and then they do nothing with it. So whenever someone asks me for advice, I always say the same thing: "Just do it." The problem has been that they mostly don't get what they need to do.

Life's not a spectator sport. You can watch your whole life fly by if you're not aware of it. So I say "Just do it," preferably right now!

Want to go the a gym? *Just do it!*

Want to drop out of college? *Just do it!*

Want to travel around the world? ***Just do it!***

...just make sure you do stuff that actually puts you in a better position than you were before. That's sort of important.

23. SNOOZING MEANS LOSING

You have a fight ahead of you as soon as the alarm clock goes off in the morning, but a lot of us delay the fight by hitting the snooze button over and over again. Then we realize that we have to go to work and suddenly everything is a mad rush.

Sounds horrible, right? It actually is horrible, so why don't you change things?

You wake up as a lesser version of yourself if you keep on snoozing. I mean, you've already postponed the first fight of the day, so why would you work any harder than that throughout the day? You'll probably end up postponing every hard task ahead of you until it all becomes a giant mess.

This might sound stupid, but the way you start your day will decide how your whole day turns out. It's all about the small things in life. In fact...

24. LIFE IS ALL ABOUT THE SMALL THINGS

People always try to do big things, but the big things don't so much matter in life. The small things actually matter in life because the small things add up and they become the big things. Getting up early was one of those small things that, when combined with other small things in your life, can lead to a real big thing, like opening your first business or changing your whole life's direction.

Constantly doing the right thing will turn you into a better person. Those things don't seem big at the moment, but they end up being the big things. Getting up early every single day, going to the gym, eating healthy, saying no to bad influences.... All those things make sure that you turn into a more disciplined person over time.

Pay attention to the small things because they really matter. How you spend today will probably give you a good indication of how you'll spend the rest of your life.

25. I WANT TO HUG EVERYBODY WHO HAS EVER HURT ME

Who wouldn't ? But would it really make any difference? Any sense?

Revenge isn't the solution. That's the easy way out. Most of these people will never understand how they've hurt you, but they can teach you a lesson about yourself. All the people who've hurt me have actually turned me into a better person - and they don't even get it! That's why I just want to hug them and say thank you. Why would I be mad at people who turn me into a better person? That would be stupid right?

Four years after my breakup, I thanked my ex and she'll probably never totally understand why I thanked her. She was the drop that spilled the cup. Without her, I wouldn't be where I am today, and I am legitimately thankful to her for that.

26. DON'T GET BITTER! GET BETTER!

Two people can face the same situation, and one can become bitter, and one become better. Some people just have to change their way of looking at certain things. To this day, I treat every new adversity that I face as a blessing in disguise. Adversity makes me better.

Many seem to break and get bitter, but that's a dangerous attitude to have. How long can you live like this before you break yourself? How much more bitterness can you and your environment endure?

Next time you feel bitter, ask yourself the following:

"Isn't this setback a blessing in disguise? Isn't there a lesson here that can make me better?"

27. THERE'S ONLY ONE OPPONENT THAT I NEED TO BEAT. I'M LOOKING AT HIM IN THE MIRROR.

People will always try to compare themselves to others. I once had a guy contact me via Instagram. He told me that he was living his life a lot like I was. I was flattered, of course, but I don't aim to compare myself to someone else. I just want to beat the person that I was yesterday. I want to go to bed and be 1% better.

This is what most people miss. They always compare themselves to others and use this to measure their success in life. This is a bit weird to me. You can only be you, so how can you use another person's unique experience like an indicator for yours?

28. HUMANITY IS THE ONLY SPECIES ON THIS ENTIRE PLANET WITH SELF- DESTRUCTIVE BEHAVIOR

J ust look at how we all live these days. Some people don't even care about their health, which is crazy if you ask me. I once met a guy who never drank water. He was always drinking energy drinks and soda, and eating fast food or other unhealthy stuff. After a while, he revealed to me that his liver wasn't working properly anymore because of his lifestyle.

I was curious why he kept living like this, to be honest, so I asked him. Turns out that he assumed that he would get a donor liver when his failed. He'd guessed he would probably live on like that with his new liver.

This is sad, right? Well, the same goes for people who are extremely overweight or enduring health issues due to unhealthy lifestyles. You won't live forever, so why don't you act a little bit more responsible, huh? Life is too beautiful to be thrown away like that.

29. YOU'RE NOT TIRED, YOU'RE JUST UNINSPIRED

I know some people who feel tired all the time. Certainly you must know a few, too. I think this means that they're either really sick... or just bored and uninspired.

The feeling of boredom will wear you out all the time. Just look at how you feel after you've playing sports. It's a much different kind of fatigue than when you're completely bored by your job. That's an exhausting and unhappy kind of fatigue. The same goes for when you watch tons of television. It's not really an activity that makes you happy, is it?

Stop doing things that make you tired in the wrong way. Make sure that you're actually doing things that energize you!

30. YOU CAN READ 500 BLOGS AND STILL ACHIEVE NOTHING

This is a reference to people who keep on reading things in order to figure life out. Sometimes you just have to start and adjust along the way.

I had a karate background when I started training MMA and everybody was mocking me at my old gym. They all assumed that karate wouldn't work because that was what had been written on the Internet. I just adjusted my style while still using karate techniques. The main thing that they should have realized is that for many parts of life, you can only know what works and what doesn't work until you've tried it yourself.

Other people just keep on researching on how to do a certain things. Just do what you want to do and make sure that reading doesn't become a form of procrastination.

31. I DON'T GO WITH THE FLOW. I FLOW WITH THE GO.

People who go with the flow can have a "whatever happens, happens" attitude. I call these people the victims of life. Something happens and they just go with the flow. They accept it, but do nothing about it otherwise.

That's not how you should approach life. You should flow with the go. This means that you work with what you've got and make the most out of it. You're adaptable to the situation and turn shit into sugar. Bruce Lee referred to this as "being like water."

32. REALITY SHOWS ARE JUST A WAY TO ESCAPE FROM YOUR OWN PROBLEMS

A lot of people like to watch reality shows these days. They basically envy others who've got nothing to offer.

This is another way that people like to compare themselves with others. They compare themselves to people who're doing worse than them and then comfort themselves. They'll be like, "See? My life isn't that bad."

But in this way, you're completely neglecting your own problems. You're avoiding the issue and this will catch up with you overtime. You either make a change or keep on lowering your standards. It's one or the other.

33. MY WAY IS A WAY, NOT THE WAY

Sometimes we force others to do things our way. But do we really have to do things like everybody else does them?

I always wanted to inspire people with my blog by sharing my struggles in life, but for some reason people started doing what I was doing. They started copying me and that's what I wanted to avoid.

The whole message behind my blog was simple: I changed my life and you can do it if I could do it. That was all there was to it. Sure, you can use my methods, but there are more ways that lead to Rome.

34. (NEVER) SAY THANK YOU TO THE PEOPLE WHO'VE HURT YOU

Remember that I once said thank you to an ex? That didn't turn out great because she didn't get it. It was a painful conversation, to be honest.

The problem was that I had changed too much and I now think that she hadn't. This is just an assumption, though, and not the objective truth. She called me a guru, asked me if I was on drugs, and so on.

Anyways, the people who've hurt you and actually caused to you to make a change probably won't get it, either. So it's best to let it go and be grateful for the lesson. Never share it with those people. Trust me, this conversation can get really weird.

I've found the humor in the situation now, laughing about it many times afterwards and probably many more times to come. But there's always one person that hurt you the worst. I still think you should thank that person. Like I said, I don't regret this action and I would do it again given the opportunity.

35. BE EGO-LESS WITH AN EGO

There are tons of books and blogs that talk about why you shouldn't have a big ego; even I have written multiple times about on the subject.

When I wrote about it, I meant "ego" in a bad way. Some people just have this giant ego about themselves without actually having accomplishing much of importance in their lives. They often link their ego to something else, like their body or car, and show it off for all to see. That's a bad ego.

Having a good ego means that you want to be the best and are willing to work for it. You don't want to be second or third, because you want to be first.

It's a relentless drive that most people don't quite understand, but look at all top competitors in their respective fields. They all have a powerful and healthy ego, even though you'll like some more than others. Some might overdo it a bit, but they're still at the top and you're just hating on them.

You need an ego to compete because losing hurts the ego and makes you work even harder the next time. People who're ego-less are happy even if they finish last. The choice is yours.

36. EAT YOUR LOSS, COME BACK LIKE A BOSS

I once entered a grappling tournament. My first opponent was a solid wrestler. We were fighting no- gi, so I had an advantage here because he wasn't as familiar with the grips. I had him in a triangle submission after 30 seconds but couldn't tap him. I basically dominated the fight and was nicely ahead on the scorecards.

However, I didn't pay any attention to those scorecards; I wanted to tap him. Eventually we got into a scramble in which, right before the bell, my opponent got a hold of me and made a last ditch effort to submit me – and it worked.

I was really pissed after that loss. It took me some time to resolve that within myself and accept that loss. But once I did, I ate the loss like a boss. I learned all I could from it and moved on. Now I have a chain of submissions ready to use in any position.

That loss made me a way better fighter. He was a good opponent and I thank him for that. I really hope he and I will meet again in a grappling tournament some day. Things might end

Alex De Wilde

up different that time.

37. YOU CAN SEE BUT BE BLIND. YOU CAN HEAR BUT BE DEAF. YOU CAN BE ALIVE YET COMPLETELY DEAD.

This quote is a reference to how most people live their lives. They see that they're doing the wrong things, but they keep on doing them. Or they see people who put in all the work and still call them "lucky" when they succeed.

Others tell them that they're not on the right path, but these people completely ignore the advice and go out to find others who screw up just as much. Some people are alive, but they never live their lives. So many people are just doing what they're told to do. They're blind and deaf without even realizing it.

Life gives you signs that indicate if you're on the right track or not. Take a good look at these signs. Listen to what life is telling you. I didn't listen when I first burned out, but I did listen when I was facing my second – depressed and on the verge of ending my life.

38. STOP LOOKING AND YOU'LL FIND WHAT YOU'VE BEEN LOOKING FOR ALL ALONG

Have you ever lost your keys or your earphones? Isn't it weird how sometimes you'll tear the house apart trying to find them only to see they're right where you left them?

Everybody has lost something in their life. Most people turn the whole house upside down to find that lost object. We're all guilty of this. But think of all the work you put into ruining your house. We turn things into a mess and have more work afterwards.

Eventually you'll find what you lost when you're not looking for it. That's how it goes with most things in life. I met my ex-girlfriend by looking right in front of me. There was no Tinder involved. I found myself again, but I was never looking to find myself in the first place. Suddenly I realized how inner peace felt and I wasn't even looking for it.

The main point here is that you can chase things your whole life, and it's exhausting, and it's frustrating because it'll always run away. But it might actually chase you when you stop chasing it. Don't look and you'll find what you want.

39. POSITIVE EMOTIONS ARE JUST AS DANGEROUS AS NEGATIVE ONES

Positive emotions are just as dangerous as negative ones, except we're just not aware of it because you can't sell anti-positivity pills so well.

Positive feelings might be fun, but they might delude you. Sometimes we're so caught up in the fact that life is going great that we lose all sense of reality. We basically set ourselves up to get hit by adversity or failure way harder than we should. Positive feelings can even make you reckless and make you dig your own grave.

This reminds me of a job interview that I once had. It was going great and I really felt it within my grasp. It was great until the guy asked me where I saw myself in five years. I told him that I was aiming for a manager spot in the company. The interviewer was, in fact, the manager and he had no intention of leaving that spot. It shouldn't be a surprise that I didn't get the job.

40. YOU HAVE FREE WILL, BUT YOUR FATE IS DETERMINED

You have free will - there's no doubt about that. In the end, you have the capability to make or break your life, but I'm pretty sure that most people aren't aware of this. They abuse their free will and think that life is unfair when they're about to face the consequences.

You can do whatever you want, but your fate is determined. You are going to die one day and you don't know when. The only problem is that some actions based on free will might make sure that you meet your determined fate a little sooner than anticipated.

Reflect on this because it might save your life one day.

41. THERE'S ONLY ONE WAY TO LEAVE A LEGACY

The only way to leave a legacy in this world is by having kids. That's the only way to make sure that everything you've earned and learned lives on in this world. People often think that starting a company, blog or being an athlete leaves a legacy, but all those things disappear. They don't remain.

We all know Muhammed Ali, but we only know him as the greatest boxer of all time. His children carry out his legacy, which is charity work. So think about having children. They're the only way to make sure that your legacy lives on. Just make sure that you don't have kids too soon because that might ruin the legacy altogether.

42. PEOPLE WHO DON'T BETTER THEMSELVES BECOME PARENTS FROM BOOKS ON THE SHELVES.

Most people never change; they simply don't learn lessons.

All of a sudden, people arrive in their mid-twenties and decide to have children because that's everyone else is doing. This works out for some, but they are mostly high-level athletes or people with a lot of life experience. I'm in my mid-twenties now and I don't want kids before I'm in my thirties, to be honest. I feel that I still have a lot to learn and don't want to become one of the parents who raises his kids without proper norms and values.

My kids should be able to do better than me when they get older because they'll get a tons of life experience right from me and my future wife to work with. They won't get the latest update about some reality show. Nobody gets better by watching and talking about those.

43. YOU'LL ALWAYS BE A PRODUCT OF YOUR ENVIRONMENT, SO MAKE SURE THAT YOU'RE A QUALITY PRODUCT

Somebody once conducted a study and found that most people who were in prison had been told, at one point or another in their life, that they would end up in prison eventually. It was a self-fulfilling prophecy.

I had heard of stuff like this when I was younger. My parents always told me that I was different and being different was bad. They told me that I would end up in prison because I didn't like rules, or that maybe I'd end up burning our house down because I was intrigued by fire when I was younger, or that I would end up homeless under a bridge because I didn't like school...

There was a lot more than that, but the main takeaway here is that you shouldn't listen to those things. You are the master of your own fate, so make sure that you create a better life for yourself. The fact that everybody thinks I'm a loser because I dropped out of college makes me work harder. I don't give in to other people's predictions and neither should you!

44. THE SHOW MUST GO ON

This is something I have heard many times from one of my training partners. He doesn't have social media besides Facebook to be able to talk to some friends in his home country, so we started talking about that. I soon realized that we had the same opinion about the whole social media hype these days.

A lot of people are so caught up in trying to convince the world that they're so perfect that they end up stuck in an unrealistic world. There is no such thing as perfection, but they still like to pretend there is.

So it's like my training partners said: the show must go on. You are what you repeatedly do, so don't do useless things because… well, it's pretty self-explanatory.

Do things that make you better because those will add up in the long run.

You are what you repeatedly do so, don't do useless things because you'll end up feeling useless. It's really that simple, but most have trouble acknowledging this.

45. IT'S PERFECTLY OK TO BE IMPERFECT

I think this is one of my key secrets as to why I'm able to do things for such a long period of time. I'm just able to accept the fact that I'm never going to be perfect at whatever I'm doing.

So many people start eating healthy and quit the second they eat something unhealthy. They always give up as soon as they "fail" or face an obstacle. Those people don't get that it's OK to mess up from time to time.

This morning, it took me 45 minutes to get out of bed. I meditated and somehow laid back down. That didn't ruin the rest of the day. I still did everything that I had planned to do. Some people skip the plan when they miss out on a part of the plan. I stick to the plan even if I have messed up a bit.

So yes, I'll eat a healthy lunch and dinner even when my breakfast wasn't so good for my body. One bird doesn't make the summer just as one unhealthy meal doesn't ruin your diet.

46. YOUR MIND IS A TOOL. IT CAN BE USED FOR SELF-DESTRUCTION.

Your mind is a tool that you should use to your own advantage because you're in serious trouble when it turns itself against you.

I still remember that my mind wasn't exactly my best friend during my depression. My mind was working against me instead of for me. It was filled with negative thoughts, insecurities, anxiety, depressing feelings, and so on. It even got me to the point where I was really going to kill myself.

Luckily for me, I eventually learned about the power of the mind and realized what a powerful tool I had in my possession. Now it's working for me instead of against me. I'm not claiming that I never face negative feelings, but they're not around 100% of the time anymore and I'm able to cope with them a lot better now when they pop up.

47. A LOT OF GUYS LIKE CLINGY GIRLS UNTIL THEY GET CHEATED ON

I once dated a clingy girl. I had the feeling that she was madly in love after the first date. After that date, she wanted to join me on a trip to Stockholm. She even claimed that she wouldn't survive if I didn't return from Stockholm because I really wanted to stay there. It was horrible to be honest and a giant turn-off. So guess what happened? She just took off with the very next guy who gave her attention.

These kinds of relationships might all seem fun at first because it's new, but this will turn into a giant nightmare. Clingy people want attention all the time, even years down the road. So guess what happens when you're giving them less and less attention? They'll cheat on you with another guy who's giving them a lot of attention.

Avoid clingy people, period.

48. PROGRESS EQUALS LIFE, STAGNATION EQUALS DEATH

You have to make sure that you're always progressing in life. That's what actually makes certain that you're alive. You're dead as soon as stagnation sets in.

Remember when I talked about the fact that you could be alive but dead? This is what I meant. You can be breathing and walking this earth yet completely death inside. Some people just go backwards in life at a certain point.

This can happen from the moment that you get comfortable and let yourself go. So make sure that you progress in life. Eat healthy, read books, talk about life, lift, do combat sports, and so on. Always make sure that you're progressing because life ends when you stagnate.

49. BE SELFISH IN A GOOD WAY. IT'S SAFE TO SAY THAT LIFE IS BETTER THAT WAY.

A lot of guys exhibit selfish behavior and they genuinely don't care about others. This is being selfish in a bad way because they'll even hurt people in the process.

But you can also be selfish in a good way, too. What I mean by this is that you priorities come first. This means that I'm not going to skip my MMA session at night for a date. We can meet before or after the session, but I won't skip it. Priorities come first.

A lot of people don't seem to get this and call me a jerk, but I have stuff to do as well. You can't always be available 24/7 for other people. Sometimes you have to be able to say "no, not now but we can do it in an hour."

My goals in life come first and everything else is secondary.

50. SOMETIMES YOU HAVE TO SPEND TIME ON YOURSELF TO REALIZE HOW HAPPY AND BLESSED YOU REALLY ARE

I'll never forget this day. It was a Sunday and I had an off day. I wanted to go for a walk in nature, but I didn't feel like it when I was driving to the park. I even felt a little bit frustrated because I was still single and didn't really see any progress on that matter. This all changed as soon as I got to the park. I suddenly realized how blessed and happy I really was. I just wandered around in the park for two hours and returned home with a big smile on my face.

I had a similar experience when I traveled to Stockholm. The only difference was that I wasn't feeling frustrated I was really happy, but I didn't realize how happy I really was until I was there. Traveling alone was an eye-opening experience for sure. That's when I realized how truly blessed I really am.

51. THE FEELING OF FRUSTRATION IS AN OPPORTUNITY TO CHANGE. USE IT WISELY.

I know a guy who worked as a truck driver for a while. He had to work eight hours a day, according to his contract, but it didn't turn out like this. He was doing shifts of 14 to 16 hours a day and had to skip training sessions on the weekend because he was so exhausted. He complained about it, of course, but he didn't change anything about it. Eventually he even had to work a couple of weekends in a row.

The unhappy feelings made him so frustrated because he constantly skipped the gym, didn't feel great, and his health was suddenly on the line because he found himself waking up with highly elevated heart beats. The next day, he went to his boss and explained that he wanted to quit. This infuriated his boss, which was the straw that broke the camel's back for my friend.

He did his time, worked there for another month and, despite his boss returning with a promotion offer, he turned it down and quit anyway. His frustration informed him wisely on the matter, I think.

52. WASTING ENERGY ON NEGATIVE THOUGHTS WILL

COMPLETELY EXHAUST YOU

Y ou know what's a big waste of time? Worrying. I once went through a period of extreme worry and it really overworked me. Your mind really is a tool and for me it became a tool of self-destruction.

I took a week off training and eventually realized that I need to make a choice to end this cycle of worry. I eventually made the right choice for my life. I needed a week to realize this, but now I know that worrying only makes you sick and tired. Nobody wants to be sick or tired, right? Just make the right decision and make sure that you don't spend hours and hours overthinking a certain matter.

53. PURPOSE GIVES MEANING TO LIFE

There's a trick that I use whenever I feel down, tired or whenever I'm in a lesser state of mind.

I take out a piece of paper and write down my life's purpose. I just write whatever I want to achieve. For example: "I have finished this ebook with 365 chapters by 21/12/2018." In this way, it's written like I've already accomplished it. The list was short in the beginning, but I've got 50 goals for now and I've even achieved some of them already.

Sometimes you've got to remind yourself that you're on this earth with a purpose, but you have to decide what that purpose is. Just make sure that it makes you happy and energized. I mean, who wouldn't want to wake up first thing in the morning knowing that there are goals to crush? You've suddenly got no reason to stay in bed anymore!

A purposeless life is a meaningless life.

54. NOT LIVING IN LINE WITH YOUR PURPOSE WILL MAKE YOU SICK

I got a fight offer in January. I was allowed to fight my first cage fight and would take it on four weeks' notice. The only problem was that I had to work on the day of the event, so I asked my boss permission to fight. She said I couldn't. I read this quote that got me thinking:

"Opportunities are like buses; there's always another one coming."

I knew this at the time, but I was pissed, no doubt about it. I got sick not much later. I was extremely tired and I couldn't recover from training or anything at all, really. (Search Google for "Zero To Alpha Pandora's Box" for the full story.) Nothing seemed to help and I only got better when I realized that I hadn't been living in line with my real goal.

I was on the mat the very next day and I was full of energy again. Nobody understood what had happened, but I did. Purpose is like a magnet: you can try to walk away, but you'll always be drawn back to it.

55. PEOPLE WHO'RE UNHAPPILY SINGLE MAINLY DON'T KNOW HOW TO USE THEIR TIME WISELY

There are a lot of unhappy singles these days. It's OK to feel alone from time to time; it can happen to anybody. But you shouldn't be dependent on another person when it comes to your happiness. This is the number-one mistake we can make because how can we expect to make someone else happy if we can't make ourselves happy?

Remember when we talked about purpose? People who call themselves "unhappy singles" have no purpose in life. They just drift around and hope to meet somebody new soon because they can't stand to live like this, alone. This mostly results in very toxic relationships.

So make sure that you've got a purpose in life. You'll be amazed at how confident and happy you become just by writing down and following your life's purpose.

56. FOLLOW YOUR GUT AND YOU WON'T GET STUCK IN A RUT

You know what happened when I didn't follow my gut feeling in life? I just ended up doing worse than I did before. I was way unhappier just because I did the opposite of what my gut was telling me to do. Your gut feeling is trying to tell you something, so try to listen to it.

The last girl that I dated seemed like trouble from the start, and I was right, but I didn't listen to my gut feeling. It took me another date to finally pull the plug. My gut has never let me down from that day on, so I keep on listening to it.

How about you? Are you listening to your gut feeling or ignoring it completely? Maybe you should spend some time on your own to listen to your gut feeling. It might tell you a lot more about your current situation than you think you know.

57. SUFFERING IS A CHOICE

There are exceptions to the rule, of course, but suffering is most of the time a choice. We all suffer in life because life throws random problems at us from time to time, but you choose how you deal with them.

A lot of people seem to suffer for a longer period of time over things that shouldn't matter that much. They turn the small things into the big things and start thinking about it all the time. Most of those things are actually not such a big deal.

I mean, remember your first real breakup? Hurt like hell, didn't it? But by the next time it happens (and it will), you realize that it's actually not that bad and you move on a lot quicker.

You can cry and feel bad about certain events, but they've happened. Learn to deal with them because you'll suffer a lot more if you're convincing yourself that you can change things that've happened.

58. CORNY QUOTES ARE REALLY CORNY, BUT THEY CAN BE 100% TRUE

People like to throw around quotes in a mocking way, but there's a lot of truth in them. Stuff like, "If you can dream it, you can do it" is actually true. People just don't take them so seriously anymore because they're thrown around so easily.

I once heard a very close-minded person share a quote about the fact that you should be open-minded. I was surprised by it, to be honest, but maybe that person had changed. Unfortunately, that was not the case. Later, I heard that the person mocked the quote and called it "a dumb, corny quote that [he] posted to get a ton of likes."

The plan worked, and it worked again when that person shared another great quote about hard work. Too bad that person never worked hard.

"Dream, believe, achieve." It's corny, but corny works. How about you?

59. MY STUMBLING STONE IS MY STEPPING STONE, TOO

This refers to the idea that "the obstacle is the way."

I injured myself in sparring the day before I started writing this book. I hit an elbow with my knee in sparring and couldn't continue. I was devastated at first because I was on a roll, but I then realized that it gave me a lot of time to write. My goal was to have 50 chapters by the end of the first week, but I had 50 chapters after just two writing sessions. I eventually got more than 100 quotes finished by the end of the week, which made me extremely happy.

You see, I could have felt sorry for myself and watched television all night, but I decided to make the most of this injury and get more writing in. The injury wasn't serious, so I only missed two training sessions, but I did have almost half of this book already written by the time I went back.

60. LEARN TO VALUE YOUR TIME OR SOMEBODY ELSE WILL TEACH YOU

I once packed a lunch and went to the city to get some writing done. I was eating in a park while I saw an old friend. She came up and starting talking. Eventually, a friend of hers joined as well. I assumed that they were going to leave because they wanted to go shopping, but they stayed because I was pretty interesting to them. I was the guy who didn't give a shit about his job and focused on other things.

I quickly realized that they were either going to join me or I was never leaving this park. So I ate my lunch and told them that I had to go because I had to get some work in. They were completely surprised because not a lot of people work on a sunny Saturday afternoon.

I realized that they just had agreed to meet up to kill time, but I had stuff to do. I had goals to crush. Learn to value your time or somebody else will make you value it.

61. MO' MONEY, MO' PROBLEMS. MO' TIME, MO' MONEY.

I once had to work three weeks in a row, but six days of that period would be paid in cash due to legal issues... or I could take a vacation. I ended up taking the vacation while others I worked with took the money. They eventually got sick and were exhausted (go figure), plus they blew all their new wealth.

Me, I traveled for 10 days in Stockholm and I made my first real amount of money during that trip via my blog. I just used the time to learn new things and live my life.

This goes back to the previous saying: "Value your time or somebody else will make you value it." Your boss doesn't care what you do, but they'll gladly pay you the money because they know you need the money. My boss was even surprised that I didn't take the money. Funny, right? It was the best decision of my life! I'm still glad that I didn't take the money. I ended up with fewer problems and more money.

62. YOU DON'T NEED PERMISSION. GO FUCKING GET IT!

It took me a while to figure this one out. We're conditioned to constantly ask for permission from other people like our teachers, parents and authorities, but they might not agree with your views on the world. Nobody supported me when I dropped out of college. People claimed that it was the dumbest thing that I could do. Turns out that it was the best thing I could have done.

It's my life. I take responsibility for my actions, failures and mistakes. I don't need anybody to constantly tell me what to do and you don't need it either. Do what you want in life but make sure that you go all in. Don't blame others for your mistakes. Don't start to hate on the system. You took a decision and now you better make it work.

So repeat this every single day: "I don't need permission. I'm going to fucking get it!"

63. THE WAY YOU VIEW THE WORLD SAYS A LOT ABOUT YOU

I once assumed that I needed to travel to see beautiful things in the world. That was the main reason I always wanted to leave Belgium. I felt like I was missing so many beautiful things abroad. I also noticed that a lot of other people share this opinion.

At some point, I started to appreciate nature here and it's not because nature changed so drastically or anything. It was me. I changed as a person. I became a better and more joyful person and saw the beauty in life that I'd seen to miss out on all these years.

Rule of thumb: people who don't appreciate nature are lost in life. I once met a person who mocked me because I was talking about a beautiful sky that I had seen. The only things she cared about was drama, gossip and social media attention. Needless to say, she wasn't really happy.

64. THE GARDEN ANALOGY, LIFE & THE WORLD

Imagine that the world is like a beautiful garden. The most beautiful garden that you've ever seen. But sometimes weeds will pop up in this garden. So what do you do when this happens? Focus on the weeds and claim that the garden is completely ruined? Or do you trim the weeds and restore order in the garden? It's up to you. The same goes for when you think about life.

So many people claim that life sucks, but it doesn't. Life is beautiful if you don't lose sight of the whole garden. Sure, you'll face things like failure, adversit, things that you don't deserve, and so on. But shouldn't you trim the weeds and restore the garden to its beauty? Stuff to reflect on, right?

It's either get bitter or get better. The garden will always stay the same. It's just up to you to make a difference and change your view on the whole matter.

65. THE BEST PIECE OF ADVICE FOR YOUR YOUNGER SELF

W hat's the best piece of advice that you would give your younger self? Someone recently asked me this question and I seriously had to think hard to provide a good answer.

The answer was extremely short: NOTHING.

I wouldn't give myself advice because every single event from the past made me to who I am today. I'm happy with the results, so why would I try to change it? Good question, right?

Most people would write down pages of advice because they can't live with the outcome of their actions. But it's not too late to change things around. Why don't you learn from your past and make sure that you've got a better future?

I'm sure about one thing: I would take a beach chair and some popcorn with me if time travel does exist. I would sit down and laugh at the things that I did wrong in the past. Sometimes you just need to get older and wiser to realize that you made some mistakes in the past. The past doesn't predict the future, though.

66. LIVE IN THE NOW. LEARN FROM THE PAST. THINK ABOUT THE FUTURE.

A lot of books wll tell you to live in the now or be in the now. That's great and all, but how can you learn from the past if you live in the now? The past doesn't exist in the now. How can you plan for the future if you don't think about the future? You don't really think about the future in the now because the future isn't in the now.

I completely agree that you should live in the now as much as possible, but I learned that I best learn lessons after something critical happens (which can be days after the event). Sometimes I learn the lesson almost immediately. It depends on the situation, I guess. And I always plan for the future at least once a week because I work in the now to get a better future. You can't work towards a future goal if you don't have one.

So learn from the past, live in the now and plan for the future. Only dogs live constantly in the now and I've never seen a millionaire dog.

67. THE BEST TIME TO START IS RIGHT NOW AND THE SECOND BEST TIME IS RIGHT NOW, TOO

This quote was a little confusing to some, but it's pretty simple. The best time to start is "right now" and the second best time is right now, as well. You have to start now and if you wait, well, you have to start right now, too!

I'm just playing with time in this quote. The first now is right now, but I'm considering the fact that you might wait. What happens if you wait? Well, that right now is gone because you've waited. That means that the second best time to start is right now. Because the second right now is happening at that particular moment.

Are you starting to get it? You should just start right now and don't give a damn about anything else!

68. SECOND GUESSING YOURSELF IS NOT AN OPTION

I'm going to share with you a lesson that I've learned through fighting. Imagine that you and I were going to fight. Imagine that you look scary as hell (tattoos, killer face, etc.).

Now imagine that I start to second guess myself. I say stuff to myself like, "I don't know if I want to do this." Guess how that'll end. I'll lose because I'm not focused. The same goes for everything in life as well: focus is key.

It's like holding a magnifying glass. What happens if you hold a magnifying glass long enough under the sun? You start a fire.

But what happens if you constantly move it? Nothing will happen! There will be no fire.

So that's what I do when I start things. I hold the magnifying glass long enough to be able to start a fire. And not just any fire. It has to be the biggest fire the world has seen.

69. ONE THING OR NOTHING AT ALL?

I remember what happened when I started doing MMA. I was considering stopping my blog because you can only do one thing well at a time, right? But the blog still exists and I've written two books since. So what happened?

Well, I realized something. I realized the power of setting priorities. MMA is number one and everything else comes secondary. It's just that easy. I spend most of my time on training, recovery and studying the sport.

Aside from that, I realized that this is a double-edged sword. I got more followers by starting this blog, which could help me make a name for myself in MMA. Or I make a name in MMA and get more people to visit my blog because of it.

It doesn't matter how it happens. What matters is that I make it happen. So focusing on one thing might actually benefit the other. It's all about setting your priorities straight (like holding the magnifying glass in the right place.)

It's time to start a fire!

70. ENJOY THE PROCESS

Did you know that writing a book was one of my childhood dreams? Somehow I suppressed that dream and forgot about until I arrived at my early twenties.

So I wrote a book and imagined how good it would feel to finally finish this book. I mean, I had been dreaming about it since I was eight years old.

The problem was that I didn't feel what I assumed I was going to feel when I finished the book. It was fun, but not as I imagined it. The other problem that I had was that I had no clue what to do next. I really wondered what would be next now that I finally achieved what I had always wanted to achieve.

I eventually focused even more so on martial arts after that. I don't make this mistake now that I'm writing this second book. I have enjoyed every single second of my writing sessions and I already know what's next after I've released this book. It sucked at the time itself, but I learned a valuable lesson from the experience.

71. HELPING PEOPLE IS THE BEST THING THERE IS

I've had my struggles in life and I'm sure that there will be a lot more struggles in the future, but that's just a part of life. Failures come and go.

I decided to start my blog because I knew that I had a story that could have an impact on people. I just wanted to make people aware that they're not the only ones who're struggling.

Helping people is a bit selfish actually since it gives you a great feeling. It's the one of the best feelings in the world next to saying what you're going to do and actually going out and do it. My blog is full of guides which are a reflection of the struggles that I had in the past.

So what's your story? What's your impact on this world? Do you actually want to help people or do you only care about yourself? It might be time to stop being so vain and admiring yourself in the mirror all the time. Ditch that mirror and look around you. So many people need help, so go out and actually help them!

72. YOUR MIND CONTROLS YOUR BODY, NOT THE OTHER WAY AROUND

Once, before a date, I got food poisoning. The food poisoning kicked in three hours before the date, but I went anyways. She had planned out the date and I had promised to show up, so I showed up. Luckily, there wasn't a lot of eating involved, but she wanted to visit a historical building, which was epic. The only problem was that we had to climb a lot of stairs.

I remember that I was so exhausted by the time that I arrived at the top. Would I do it again? Absolutely. Do I remember a lot about the date? Not a lot, to be honest.

The same goes for fighting. Sometimes you're exhausted with only one minute to go. So that means that you'll have to push it one more minute. Or you get clipped and need to survive. There are times when you need to rest and times when you need to push on. It's up to you to learn the difference. In the end, you'll see how bad you really want it.

73. BORED? HOW CAN YOU BE BORED IN THIS DAY AND AGE?

This is something that I still don't get. People go to work and then come home and watch television until they fall asleep. There are so many people who even sleep longer during the weekends because they've got nothing going on in their lives. They don't sleep because they're really tired. They sleep because they're bored and uninspired.

I just wonder how you're able to be bored in this day and age. It's never been easier to have access to information. It's never been easier to learn new things and still you've got no clue on how you should spend your time? I know why some people don't get how they should spend their time. It's because every medium that can teach you things has a curse.

But what if the things I like doing don't make me money? More on that in the next chapter...

74. DO WHAT YOU LIKE AND FORGET ABOUT THE MONEY

E ver seen what happens when people chase money? They do jobs that they don't like. Sad, isn't it? This cannot be you. You cannot, I repeat, you *cannot* live like this.

Do something that you really like (I chose MMA and blogging) and don't worry about the money. Pick a normal job on the side for 30-40 hours a week to make sure that you can pay everything you need and see how happy you'll be.

The great thing is that there's actually a chance that you make money by doing what you actually like, so keep on doing it! This might ensure that you can stop your normal job and do whatever you like and get paid for it. A lot of people wonder what happens if it doesn't work out. Well, then you had a fulfilling time and take away a ton of life lessons to share with other people.

How do you guess that I learned so much? I focused on living live and I didn't give a single fuck about all the rest.

75. THE SUBTLE ART OF NOT GIVING A FLYING FUCK

My boss once told me, "It's like you don't care at all." This was after he had become angry because I was 15 minutes late. He just wanted to prove that he was the boss. (Fun fact: I didn't care.)

But people don't get how I'm able to be careless about so many things. The secret is that I do care about things, but only about the things that I can actually control. So I don't care if I get rejected because I'm not somebody's type; I don't care about people who hate me; I don't care about the fact that I've got an accent when I'm talking English; I don't care what's going on in our neighbors house; and so on.

There are only a few things in your life that you've got complete control over. That's your life, your actions, your attitude, your perception of things, your work ethic... The list does go on, of course. There are only a few things that you actually can control in life, so focus on those and don't give a fuck about the rest.

76. MY BIGGEST FEAR TURNS OUT TO BE MY BIGGEST MOTIVATION

I can't stand the thought of living a normal life. I just can't bring myself to call this kind of life "fulfilling." I mean, what's fulfilling about following the herd without ever wondering what you could have accomplished in life?! I don't want that and you, too, should think decide for yourself if you want it or not. Your future depends on this.

I'm just not the kind of person who can live with the fact that I have worked for the same company in the same cubical for 40 years. It sounds like absolute death to me.

I couldn't live with the fact that I have to do this and that just to fit in. Being normal doesn't really make me happy, so why would I even attempt to pretend that I like it? I don't get paid to act, so I'm not doing it.

Where are you at on this subject? Do you want to live a life like this? There's nothing wrong with it if you like it. But I suggest that you be honest with yourself about it sooner than later.

77. EVERY INNOVATOR WILL ATTRACT MORE THAN ONE HATER

My osteopath is an innovator in every way of the word. He actually cares about people and is turning science upside down. He once published an article where he completely debunked the use of painkillers. He showed that they were more harmful than beneficial.

Later that month, I had an appointment with him and I mentioned that I had read the article and really enjoyed it. He took his laptop and showed me the comment section on Facebook. There were tons of doctors who were hating on him. He didn't care at all, but that was an eye-opener for sure.

I've always liked sparring with my hands down. I'm not an innovator in that regard; most people do it. But my old trainer really hated it. He told me to keep my hands up at all times. I experimented with this in Sweden at my gym and nobody said a thing. You know why? Because I knew when to do it and when I couldn't do it.

78. MISERY LOVES SOME COMPANY IN A COMPANY

I worked at a garden center for more than a year. I absolutely hated it, but I stayed for the benefits. The boss was nice on occasion, but she could insult you out of nowhere at the drop of a hat. She did this to everybody.

I made it clear that I didn't put up with this kind of behavior. You don't insult me and act nice afterwards to get away with this behavior. It doesn't work like that.

But a lot of my co-workers did accept this behavior because she was the boss. So they complained about it from time to time. They basically complained about everything, but they never really talked about it, so nothing ever changed. It might be fun to complain about your boss at the water cooler, but nothing will change. Get away from people who act like this. They have toxic mentalities.

This is probably another reason why I didn't like normal jobs. Nobody was happy! They all complained and nothing changed.

79. FIND AN ENVIRONMENT THAT CHALLENGES YOU

I trained MMA in a gym for two years, but all the good training partners left, so I always had to restart with people. I was sick of this, so I left the gym to make sure that I kept improving my stand-up. I still went to the gym once a week to train BJJ because they were going to prepare for the Europeans. That all changed when I heard the news that they weren't competing there at all because they were too signing up.

Another one of my grappling partners left for another gym to improve his grappling. He eventually asked me to join and that's what I did. I joined him and left the other gym for good. It doesn't matter if you don't want to compete, but I want to compete, so I want to train with absolute killers who push me to the limit. What doesn't challenge you doesn't change you. Corny, but true.

Normal jobs never really challenged me, so I have never really held onto one for very long.

80. TACTICAL UNEMPLOYMENT, A.K.A. "THE SABBATICAL YEAR."

Y ou know that I'm a college dropout, but did you know that I worked for three months total during that whole year? Crazy, right? I got a lot of shit for doing this. I basically found a job rather quickly, made a lot of money and lived on that. I looked for a new job in the time between, but never really found one. They either fired me after a day or never really accepted me.

Instead I focused on martial arts, improving myself and writing my blog. This was a bad year income-wise, but there was a lot of growth, too. So it wasn't that bad after all.

I think more people should take a sabbatical because you'll learn a lot about yourself during that period. I absolutely loved that year, although I never had the intention to take a sabbatical. I just didn't want to end up in the first job that they handed to me.

So take some time off to get to know yourself. Don't listen to the others. People who judge you have never found their self in the first place.

81. YOU CAN'T DEFEAT ME, SO WHY EVEN BOTHER?

Pretty bold claim, isn't it? People always assume that it's cocky, but I don't think it is. This is an actual fact. I either win or I learn and make a comeback, but there's not a single person alive that can beat me. Try to apply this mindset as well.

Life is hard from time to time but I will not be defeated - that's it. I'd rather drop dead than give up. Some people think that I'm crazy. That's their opinion. You have to be this intense if you really want something. It's do or die. No do or try.

This is the number one reason why so many people fail, in my opinion. They'll promise to do something, but they mostly won't. It's like the guy who buys a gym membership and is already making excuses that he won't be able to make it every single day because of some weird reason. Most people basically defeat themselves before they've even started. It's sad but true.

82. PEOPLE PUT ON AN ACT DESPITE NEVER RECEIVE BEING ELIGIBLE TO WIN AN OSCAR

S ome like to act as if everything goes perfectly in their life and that's a mistake. Perfection doesn't exist. I'm not afraid to admit when I face some rough times or fucked something up. It's part of life and I embrace it.

Life is full of highs and lows, so I try to walk the middle line. Most people are living in the so-called "perfect relationship," but those are just acts. I realize now that most people have no clue about what a good relationship looks like. I know two couples who are really happy together. Maybe three.

Peoples' lives look like a dramatic TV show because they act all the time. You can't solve all your problems if you never acknowledge them. It's stupid to neglect them and even dangerous for your own mental health. So stop pretending that everything is fine. Admit your problems, because no one is giving you an Oscar for your acting.

83. THE NICE GUY WILL ALWAYS FINISH LAST BECAUSE NICE GUYS ARE ASSHOLES

The nice guy is an asshole - he just doesn't know it. Most people don't recognize this.

The nice guy is only nice to girls that are hot in his opinion. He'll help a hot girl in a certain situation, but he won't do it for a less attractive girl in that same situation. A real good guy is nice to everybody and doesn't act like a nice guy to get laid. So

Nice guys are always nice with a hidden agenda against other people. They're always trying to manipulate you, so be aware of these people. They might smile at you in the morning and stab you in the back at night.

84. THERE'S A PLACE WHERE THE FRUSTRATED PEOPLE GATHER. IT'S CALLED "THE COMMENT SECTION."

Ever seen a regular comment section on YouTube? Normally I never read those comment sections, but I used to glance at them when I was bored at work. There's a lot of hate in these comment sections and people don't seem to get that they're actually hurting others. It's easy to sit behind the computer all day and offend people, but those people are actually hiding.

I mean, what's the point of offending someone because you don't agree with them? Pretty damn stupid, isn't it? It's even extremely close-minded, in my opinion. I have one simple message for these people: get a life! I've seen some really offensive things in the YouTube comment section, things that can deeply hurt another human being.

85. YOU HAVE TWO LIVES, BUT MOST PEOPLE ONLY LIVE ONE

So I've said you've got two lives, now you're probably wondering how this plays out. Well, your second life starts when you realize, "Wow, I've only got one life."

There'll be a point in life in which you'll realize that you've got to wake up. Or you'll reach that point without realizing that you've got to wake up and then there'll be no change.

So how do you get your wake-up call? Well, you've got to step out of your comfort zone. That's where the real growth starts. That's a hard task, but you can't change your life if you're not going outside that comfort zone.

And then, something magical will happen: you'll get comfortable with the uncomfortable. You just have to do the things that you think that you can't do and control your inner bitch. You'll quickly notice that the word "impossible" is invented by your mind and other people.

You have to turn impossible into "I'm possible." So grasp the change when the wake-up call comes and start your new life.

86. BEING A LOSER TAKES ZERO EFFORT, BUT IT'S A HARD LIFE

I t's easy to be a loser, right? I mean, it requires zero effort to be one and a lot of guys live like this in this day and age. They just watch porn and YouTube all the time. They're the skinny, wannabe tough guys, but they crack as soon as get into a real fight.

These guys actually have a hard life. They're putting up an act that's getting exposed all the time, but they don't want to admit it. This is a vicious cycle. But the hardest part is that they have zero fulfilment in their lives. You can't feel fulfilled if you don't work hard, which is why these people aren't that happy at all.

It's a harsh life!

87. CONTRADICTING YOURSELF IS NOT AS BAD AS YOU MIGHT THINK

A guy once told me that it would be pretty awkward for me if I contradicted myself on my blog. I didn't really ask him why he shared this because he's not so open-minded. But I thought about his remark and I came to the conclusion that contradicting yourself over time isn't that bad.

You see, you always grow as a person or you're supposed to grow as a person, at least. So how can you hold onto the same beliefs if you keep on growing? Some beliefs might never change, but others will change drastically.

So it's actually not that bad to contradict yourself over time. The people who call you out are the ones who haven't changed and aren't smart enough to get that you've changed.

They might still have the same views as 10 years ago, but that shouldn't mean you have to. Keep evolving, keep living!

88. ARE YOU REALLY UNWORLDLY OR JUST SMARTER THAN THE OTHERS?

People like to show off with all the facts that they know about the world.

I really don't care, to be honest. I have no clue what's happening where. I have no clue who the president of France is and so on. But why would I need to know this stuff? To show off to others? That's a fools way of seeking glory.

Everybody can memorize these facts and everybody can google these facts. So why would I try to recall facts that can be googled in an instant? I seriously don't see the point in doing so. I fill my head with things that are useful. Stuff that are related to life in the larger sense or to martial arts. I just don't care about anything else and I'll google it if you really want me to answer the question.

I mean, I'm pretty sure that no successful person knows how long the longest river in the world is, but they all know how to make and keep money. Isn't that more useful?

89. YOU MIGHT LIKE TO TWERK, BUT I LOVE HARD WORK

People don't love the grind anymore these days. They're basically raised in an environment that pushes them into a comfort zone. I mean, how many people grow up without a television nowadays? We didn't have a television until I was six. But I understand that people are raised by their parents and it is this that makes them develop and keep habits. They see how their parents live and basically copy the behavior.

I was once like that, but I changed when I realized something that I really liked. Suddenly, I realized that hard work doesn't really make you tired. It energizes you in a good way.

A lot of people miss out on this experience because they start to complain about the fact that they have to put in effort before they've even started. So they half-ass it and don't feel the same as I do.

90. LEARN TO SWEAT. THE MORE YOU SWEAT, THE LUCKIER YOU GET.

Nobody is self-made even if they claim to be. Most people won't believe me, but there's not a single person in the world that has done it on his own. I had never considered the word "self-made" to describe my big change but others did. I didn't see it that way.

Arnold opened my eyes. Suddenly, I got it. We all have had help in life, but some people just don't seem to realize it. They're not grateful and that's not the right mindset. You should always be grateful no matter what.

I got help from books, friends, YouTube, and so on. People don't seem to realize that we have tons of resources for help. You can learn literally anything online these days. You didn't figure out anything and we're still claiming that we did it all on our own.

So why do people claim it? Because they've got a big ego- that's why. Some people's ego grows at the same rate as their bank account, but they'll eventually need to be humble again. Life will bring humility upon you if you're not humble in life.

91. PASSION WILL GET YOU NOWHERE IN LIFE

Have you ever heard of passion? Of course you have since it's used a lot by motivational speakers.

I don't have the intention to become a motivational speaker, but I would never talk about passion. I don't even know what it is. You can't eat it or be it. It's just an empty emotion that makes sure that you do absolutely nothing. That's what it is, nothing more and nothing less. Passion is the zero, but obsession is the alpha.

People who are passionate aren't getting anything done in a day. They do a lot, but it's all wasted time. People who are passionate seem to be afraid of acting on something that they really like.

Can you guess how many bills get payed with passion? None!

People who practice sports at a high level are obsessed, but not passionate. Guess where all the passionate people are? Those are the people who're cheering in the stadium. They know everything about the sport, but now how to play and that's why they don't get paid.

92. ONLY A FOOL WILL CHASE EVERYTHING THAT'S COOL

L et me make it clear once and for all: *forget about the excessive clubbing.* Forget about drinking and getting wasted all the time. I stopped drinking a year ago and I'm doing great.

Forget about chasing the cool because it'll make you look like a fool. And forget about chasing girls because it's just plain stupid.

I made all of these mistakes in the past and I wasn't happy. I was far from happy. Being popular wasn't cool at all. It was a lonely and depressing feeling all because I couldn't be myself.

So now you've got two options. You either learn from my mistakes or you make them and realize that I was right later. You can chase the pot of gold your entire life, but how long will it take before you realize that it is completely empty?

93. FAMOUS FOR NOTHING TO GET SHIT FOR FREE

A lot of people want free stuff, so they'll get on Instagram and try to become famous through the Internet. They spend tons of money on photoshoots or take pictures of everything they eat in the right lighting. Even people who work out take this approach. They just want to do nothing and get money for doing it.

It doesn't work that way! Well, it works, but you'll never feel fulfilled. You'll eventually feel extremely bored and feel like doing nothing.

These people's identity is bound to social media, which is pretty bad. Their ego grows as soon as their likes and followers go up. They don't realize that ego is their worst enemy. There are even people who mocked me because they were more popular on Instagram. I don't have a problem with that since I don't care about social media. I care about making a difference.

Famous for nothing to get shit for free... That ain't me.

94. LISTEN TO COMPREHEND INSTEAD OF WITH THE INTENT TO REPLY

A lot of people only listen with the intention to speak.

I met a guy like this once. We each had a date on a Friday night and the next day, he asked me how my date went. I didn't attend the date because I'd been rejected by text an hour before it even took place. So I just sent him a screen shot and told him that I had to take some time to reflect on this. I was basically saying that I didn't want to talk about it yet because I wanted to figure out what happened first.

He didn't get the message at all. He just started bragging about his dates. (Turned out he had had multiple.) The only reason that he asked about my date was so he could talk about his date. Crazy, right? I didn't even know that such people existed. So only ask questions if you're really interested in the answer. Never ask questions to make sure that you can talk about yourself.

95. THE EX-FILES: ARE YOU COMPLETELY DOOMED?

I wrote this post after I met a guy who claimed that he had found the love of this life. I met that girl and she was just like his ex but in a different body. So guess how it turned out? He just got dumped once again and didn't understand why.

The same goes for girls who "always" fall for bad boys. How unlucky can you even be? Very unlucky, right?

The reality is that dating, like everything, contains lessons. You'll keep on making the same mistakes if you don't learn these lessons or you'll settle for less.

So give yourself a reality check next time you date someone. Ask yourself what you did wrong regardless of what the other person did. For example: though she might have controlled you, you let her, so who's to blame?

Someone once told me that it takes two to tango. Learn your lessons or you'll end up doing a solo shuffle.

96. BE THE WRITER OF YOUR OWN STORY

I magine that you were the writer of your own story. You have a pen and paper, and you can start the story however you want. You're in charge.

Would you live the life that you're living now? Or would you make a drastic change? It's always different if you look at your life from a new perspective.

The fact that you can write your own story means that you're free to do whatever you want. You can do crazy things, chase dreams and so on. There are no self-imposed limits which you have in real life. All those things disappear.

So why don't you take up the pen and paper and start writing? I did this once and I quickly realized how much I really lived under my potential. I was underperforming and that's an understatement.

97. SO, TELL ME WHY ARE YOU WAITING ON THE PERFECT MONDAY?

People always have great plans when they start something new and inevitably they always want to start on Monday. I seriously don't get this.

These people mostly hype the event up and convince everybody that life will be so great after they've crushed their project. But then that particular Monday arrives and they mess up somewhere along the line. Maybe they want to start a diet but they ate unhealthily, or they want to start a blog but they didn't really write anything. So they're pissed and completely quit the project and claim that it wasn't for them. How can you know if it wasn't for you if you didn't even really try it?

Aside from that, I wonder how committed you really were. I mean, I would start right away if I really wanted something. I started training MMA on a random day in the week just because I really wanted to do it. The same goes for blogging. I just started because the perfect Monday will never arrive. It's a myth.

98. JUST ASK. BE PROACTIVE!

I needed a review team when I launched this book but there was only one single problem. I was staying in Thailand and I didn't know anybody over here yet. So I just started asking around in the Muay Thai community if people would be interested in reading my book. There were a lot of people who wanted to help me out and I got 10 in no time.

The main lesson is pretty simple here: just ask people for help if you need some. Sure some people said no but the majority didn't. They were happy to help and I would do the same for them if they'd ask me.

99. DID SOMEONE DISAPPOINT YOU OR DID YOU DO IT TO YOURSELF?

This is a great example of "expectation meets reality." I think it's safe to assume that we all have had a situation in which we assumed that we were going to nail something, then completely fucked it up and ended up devastated. Or that we didn't look forward to something and eventually actually liked it.

It doesn't really matter what happened. What matters is that we learn that our emotions can fool us. Never sell the bear's skin before you has killed the beast. So never assume that you've nailed something if you haven't even done it yet. Or don't assume that something is boring before you've done it. It's just an assumption. Learn to be present in the moment.

Don't hype yourself up. Don't delude yourself. Just do what you have to do and see what happens. You'll be crushed if it didn't go your way. Trust me on this one.

100. THE MOST POWERFUL SUPPLEMENT ON EARTH

Motivational speakers always talk about the power of the mind, and we all know why, right? Because you can achieve it if you believe it.

Over the course of the years, I've seen how powerful the mind really is. I've seen people who sneezed once and believed that they were going to get sick. Guess what happened the next day" Sure enough, they got sick. I'm not saying that you'll never get sick, but some people get sick all the time because the mind got sick before the body.

So what's the main lesson here? You should exercise you mind just like your body. A healthy body with an unhealthy mind isn't healthy. So read, meditate and take care of your mind.

Make sure that you actually have a strong mind in a strong body. "Mens sana in corpore sano." It's an old saying and so many people neglect it.

101. LEARN TO
BE ALONE

This might be me talking as an introvert, but I've learned a lot from being on my own. I've learned a lot about myself, to be honest.

People think that it's weird that I go on long walks to places I'm certain there's no wifi. I do this to make sure that I reload. Don't get me wrong: I love being around people, but it's draining as well. People need your attention, so that drains your energy.

You need to realize that there's a big difference between being alone and being lonely. People who are lonely are in pretty bad company and they don't even know it. Well, they know it, but they don't want to admit it. So they'll look for other people to hang around with to escape their own miserable faith. Their demons will catch up with them, so why not face them now while they're still small?

102. AYW: ACCESS YOUR "WHY"

Ever heard of AYW? It's forces you to answer the most difficult question that's been asked by every four-year-old ever: "Why?"

It's easy to say "that's why" and move on, but that doesn't make you a better person, does it? Sometimes we have to address our emotions and ask why we feel a certain way. Sometimes you should ask yourself why you're happy, because you have to take notes during the good and bad times in life. You need to be aware of what you do wrong and right.

Here's an example: I noticed that I always felt the urgency to spend a lot of time on my phone at my normal job and after it, too . I didn't like it, but I did it anyways. I did it until I asked myself why I did it.

Turns out that I was so bored that I need other sources to entertain me. Stuff like the news and social media. I started spending way less time on my phone as soon as I understood this. AYW could improve your life big time!

103. THE ONLY WAY TO AVOID HATERS

Some people don't like it when people start to hate on them, but it's a part of negative peoples' nature. You either deal with it or you can use this easy hack. It's possible to have zero haters in life. Sounds great, doesn't it?

But with everything good comes something bad. You'll pay the price on this one. So be sure about your decision before you move on.

Here's the only way to avoid haters: don't do anything new or interesting. Just follow the textbook and that's it. People will never hate on you, but you might never accomplish your goals, either, so is this really what you want?

Wouldn't it be better to learn to deal with haters instead of trying to avoid them? They're a necessary evil because they really can make you famous. You just don't see it yet.

104. HATERS MAKE YOU FAMOUS

D id you know that haters make you famous?

They talk about you so much that people will check you out because of them. Great, right?

Even all the hateful comments are actually a great thing. Google doesn't know the difference between a hateful comment and a supportive comment. So they'll just rank your website based on traffic, comments and so on. The more comments, the better the rankings.

So why would you bother about people who talk shit about you? They actually promote you for free. Some people even use most of their time to hate/promote others. So we should be grateful that people want to hate/promote us for free. Smart people actually make money when they're promoting others.

105. SOME PEOPLE WANT TO SEE YOU GO DOWN

I had a buddy (we're not buddies anymore) who was friends with me because he could place himself above me. He continue to try this kind of thing when I started my journey of self-improvement.

He quickly realized that it wouldn't work, so he started hating on me. He even told me in my face that he wanted to see me knocked out in my first fight. Did I take it personally? Hell no! I just learned a valuable lesson.

I realized that some people want to keep you at your old level because they don't want to improve. They want to stay the same and they want you to stay the same, as well. Pretty sad, isn't it? But I don't want to stay like I was in the past. I want to improve every single day!

Just get away from these people. They'll hate on you until you make it and then they'll kiss your ass because you're making more money than them. Sad but true, so make sure that it doesn't happen to you.

106. MINDSET HACK TO GET YOU BACK ON TRACK

I have a simple sentence that I tell myself from time to time: "I can do it if someone else can do it." I might even do it better. I'll also be the first one if nobody else has done it yet.

A lot of people label things as impossible, but what's impossible? How can you know if something is impossible if you haven't even tried yet? It's a bit weird, don't you think? Doesn't sound right if you ask me! Turn "impossible" into "I'm possible."

You would think that I'm absolutely crazy if you would hear all the goals that I've set for myself, but I'm going to do everything to make them happen. They've all been achieved before, but never by a guy from Belgium. So why couldn't I be the first one?

I'm possible and you're possible as well. 'nuff said.

107. DON'T TALK, JUST WALK

A lot of people like to make bold claims about what they're going to do. I've met a lot of self-proclaimed billionaires and athletes, but they've never even made it to training.

You know what I did when I knew what I wanted to do in life? I just showed up where I needed to be. I just started working towards my goal. I never talked about it with other people because I didn't see the point in doing so. You're trying to convince yourself that you want this, but deep down you know that you don't want to put in the work.

Start working if you really want to accomplish something. Don't make all these bold claims to people or in a comment section. They might believe you at first, but they'll see through the act after your third or fourth failed project.

People call me a walker and not a talker. I like to keep it that way. This means that they see me as someone who takes action. Strive to be the same.

108. MALE FEMINISTS ARE THE WORST

I'm all for equal rights, but I really hate some male feminists. They're basically acting like feminists just to get laid. This kind of behavior is pretty disturbing.

I have never quite understood why guys would put up an act to be liked by others. It's extremely stupid. It's this kind of pussy behavior that gives real men a bad name.

I can draw a brief conclusion if you're like that: you're a wannabe white knight and you're not going to get laid tonight.

Chew on that.

109. HEY, ALEX, ARE YOU PART OF (INSERT ANY KIND OF POPULAR MOVEMENT)?

Someone once asked me on Snapchat if I had taken "the red pill." I never heard of it, but I googled it anyways. It seemed to be some kind of men's rights movement. So no, I'm not a part of it and here's why:

In MMA there are two kinds of fighters. You have the strikers and the grapplers. They both link themselves to one aspect of the sport, which is stupid if you ask me. They neglect another part of the sport completely.

So I'll tell people that I'm a mixed martial artist if they ask me what my fighting style is. I don't neglect things and I don't link myself to movements. These movements mostly take things to the extreme and neglect things that shouldn't be neglected.

They're part of our modern-day generation, I guess. They

come and go like most overhyped things do.

110. THE POWER OF ACCEPTANCE

Remember that grappling tournament that I entered? Did you know that I didn't have a lot of stress before the match? One of my training partners, on the other hand, was about to burst a blood vessel. He was extremely stressed.

What was the difference between him and I? I had accepted the fact that a higher heart rate and so on would occur. That's just my body getting ready to fight. I had also accepted the fact that I could lose or that I could end up in bad situations, whereas he was constantly asking himself what if questions. Those "what if" questions are sometimes hard to answer if you're not actually experiencing the situation you're worrying about.

This also goes for things that happen to us. Sometimes you just have to accept the situation and "flow with the go." The event loses power over you the moment you accept it.

111. DUMB AND DUMBER

ost people stop learning as soon as they've gradu-
ated. They link pain and misery to the learning process, so they avoid it like the plague. They're conditioned in a bad way, but they're to blind to see it. They learned
something that they didn't like at all, but never took the time
to learn something that they really liked.

This enforces the fact that they will keep on hating the learning process. They just enroll in a job and only learn new stuff
that involves their job. How can you expect to become a
smarter human being when you're living like a fucking machine? Your mind is slowly put to sleep and you'll feel cheated
by life 20 years down the line.

So make sure that you don't end up like most people. Read
every single day and listen to podcasts. It doesn't matter what
you do. Just make sure that you get smarter.

112. PICK THE RIGHT WIFE FOR THE SAKE OF YOUR LIFE

Ever heard of the saying, "Behind every strong man is a strong woman"? This is true! This is what happens when yin and yang become one.

The problem is that most people just settle because they have to settle or they settle because they caught an attractive piece of meat they'd like to claim. It's sad, but this is the most common approach. Nobody likes to improve themselves, work on goals, and then meet the love of their life. That's pretty overrated apparently.

So why don't you change your approach? Why don't you work on yourself and your goals and see who you meet during that period? It might be someone extremely wonderful who builds an empire together with you! Doesn't that sound a lot better than a sexless marriage that ends with a divorce? I don't want to live like that and I can't imagine that somebody else would like it, either.

113. READ BOOKS AND FORGET ABOUT THE LOOKS

We're living in a fucked-up society these days. People are tricked into thinking that looks are everything these days, but that isn't true.

There are women these days who look like a Picasso painting instead of something else. Some even look like they're made out of plastic. It's just a layer to hide their insecurity, but it doesn't work.

Men have more beauty products than women these days. They use creams for this and that. Plastic surgery is getting extremely popular, plus I recently heard that you can get a surgery to get a bigger jawline. This is all pretty fucked-up, in my humble opinion.

Don't get me wrong; you shouldn't dress like a bum. You need to impress instead of dress. What I mean is, focus on the face. Not the body, since that's something that you can improve just by doing sports.

I'd rather have my average looks and a developed mind than

great looks and an empty head.

114. WHY DO MOST PEOPLE HAVE DRUNK PERSONALITIES?

I think that we all can agree upon the fact that some drunk personalities are more pleasant than others. Alcohol enhances what you feel but also what and who you are. So you'll turn into an asshole if you're deep down inside an asshole.

Most people aren't true to themselves and in some cases, it's for the better. Some people really step over the line when they've indulged in too much alcohol. People have the tendency to tell the truth when they've consumed too much alcohol. Those people say the things that they're afraid to say when they're sober.

Most people tend to forgive this behavior because they claim that it was the alcohol that changed them, but did it really change them?

Be realistic here: they didn't change. These people are people-pleasers when they're sober, but guess what? They don't like you. It's a cowardly way of living, in my opinion. They just blame the alcohol for being themselves.

115. PEOPLE ARE ALWAYS LOOKING FOR THE NEXT BIG THING AND THEY NEVER FIND IT

I remember someone who was determined to get popular by blogging. The blog got published, but there weren't a lot of posts. Suddenly, attention was being paid to the next big thing.

Instagram happened to be that next big thing. So all the attention went to Instagram and then it suddenly changed to YouTube until the next "big thing" pops up.

There is no next big thing. Blogging is still the future and I'm sure that you can make a lot of money through Instagram as well. The one thing that you've got to realize is that you've got to put in the work and keep on going. You can set up five things and never achieve a single one.

I have a blog, a podcast and a YouTube channel, but I don't

abandon anything. The podcast and the YouTube channel are there to support the blog. I don't look for the next big thing. I turn my blog into the next big thing.

116. THE YEAR OF THE ALPHA

I remember I claimed once that 2018 would be my year, but I had to face one setback after the other. It was a challenging year for sure. I'm grateful that it happened because it shaped me as a person even more.

The depression made me change my life; the years after that were just trial and error. Now I know who I really am. It's like I claim in the blog: my year started on the first of November. I'm two months ahead of the game.

Some people thought that this was arrogance, but it's not. I embraced all the obstacles and got past them one by one. Those people didn't see or get what I went through. But I know why they don't get it. They don't get it because they've never had such a life-changing year. They've basically avoided it and that's why they still face the same problems.

117. BECOME TOUGHER WITH THIS EASY GUIDE

People who know me always claim that I'm tough as nails, but did you know that I wasn't always like this? In fact, I used to be a very weak person. I would shy away from basically every challenge that I had in life.

So you're probably wondering what changed. My attitude and actions changed. I started to take the right actions (i.e. the actions that turn you into a strong person.) Because you can claim that you're tough all you want until you really get tested. Your reaction in that situation will be based on all the small actions that you took in life. In the end, it's all about the small details, remember?

So take a closer look at your past actions. I used to blame people, gossip, hate on successful people and so on. I was weak until I decided to be strong. You don't decide to be weak, but you can decide to be strong. Start being strong today.

118. THE MORNING PERSON: IS IT AN OVERHYPED MYTH?

People claim that there are two kinds of people. You're either a morning person or a night owl. I say there are two kinds of people: the ones who take action and the ones who don't.

I noticed that people who like to sleep in are mostly uninspired people who have no clue on how they should spend their time. People who love to be active, on the other hand, get up earlier because they actually love to get the day started. So tell me, are you really tired or just uninspired?

119. WHY YOU SHOULD NEVER WATCH THE NEWS

I 'll never forget a certain quote from a book. It was from a guy who had worked for a newspaper. His job was to look for the most horrible news out there. He eventually quit his job and never watched the news again, and you shouldn't watch it either.

I mean, how many people do you know that are completely joyful after watching the news? Don't get me wrong, you should be aware of the horrible things that happen in this world.

However, you should also be aware of the fact that the news will never show all the beautiful things in life. That's probably because the ratings would be a lot lower. It's in human nature to love drama, I guess. Just use your time wisely.

Besides, I'm always in the gym when the news is about to air. How about you?

120. HOLDING GRUDGES DOESN'T SOLVE JACK SHIT

A lot of people have the tendency to hold grudges these days. This is crazy if you ask me. They want the other person to be unlucky while they're constantly poisoning their mind.

Why are you holding grudges towards someone else? Do you even know why? Don't you have better things to do? I mean, there's nothing more destructive than holding a grudge.

Nobody cares about the fact that you're holding grudges, either. Well, nobody besides you, of course. The person you hate won't even realize that you're hating them. Most people have no clue what they did wrong. They'll probably laugh at it and ask you if you're still mad about something they did. They don't consider it a big deal, but you will. You see your thinking is simply ego-driven. They'll be partying while you're still hating. Just think about that!

121. EVERYTHING HAS ALREADY BEEN WRITTEN BEFORE

Hard to believe, huh? But you're still reading this book. There is so much wisdom in books, but most people neglect it. They read the stuff that's been written somewhere else.

Blogs about how to be a good person are extremely popular, but do we really need to read this? Don't we know how to be good people? There's a big chance that you've read things in my book that've been written elsewhere before. I just write them with a touch of my personality, which makes it so different from the rest. This is how all writing is done!

Blogs wouldn't exist if people constantly did the right thing. It's a good thing that people don't always do the right thing, otherwise my blog wouldn't have ever existed in the first place.

122. NEVER TAKE A CHEAT DAY ON A WORK DAY

I remember this day like it was yesterday. I had finished working at 3 P.M. and was going to write and train in the afternoon. At night, I ate pizza, but I ate a little earlier because I had training. I got nothing done after I finished that pizza and eventually even skipped training.

I ate more than the pizza, of course, but there is a great lesson to be learned here. Put fuel in your body if you're looking to work or train. There are people who're able to do it, but I can't. My body just doesn't like it that much. That's why I mostly cheat on my off days.

It doesn't really matter that I don't feel like working then since I don't have to at all. So be strategic with what you put in your body and when.

123. THERE ARE 2 SIDES TO EVERY STORY

I remember my first MMA coach. He was always talking about how some people disrespected him and how he always demanded respect. You believe everything he says at first, of course, because you only hear one side of the story.

That all changed when I started to mature and eventually met some people who had trained at my old gym. They told me why they left, but they did it in a respectful manner and they all gave the same reasons. Aside from that, those were the reasons why I wanted to leave as well. The old trainer always talked about them as if they left because they weren't good enough, but I quickly realized that they left to actually get better.

So never, ever only listen to one side of the story, because you might be starting at the wrong end of it.

124. PEOPLE ALWAYS CLAIM THAT THEY WANT THE BEST FOR YOU

I got more active on social media after I left my first gym. It was just a coincidence. But I let the world know who I really was. I didn't care about the worlds opinion of me because I was really me and I was happier now because I was training at a new and better gym.

I didn't have any problems with my old trainer until he posted a message on his Instagram. He put this on his story: "You look great, but you can't FIGHT." I knew it was aimed at me. He knew that I was getting better at my new gym and couldn't handle it. It was pretty disgusting and childish, in my opinion.

I didn't react to it, but I knew with what kind of person I was dealing right now. I just knew that I was never going to set a foot in that gym again.

125. HOW TO DEAL WITH INTERNET HATERS

R emember that my trainer tried to hate on me online? Well, he basically gave me a compliment first by talking about my looks.

At first, I was going to react to it. Maybe something like, "thanks for letting me know you think I'm handsome!" But then I realized that that might have been the thing that he actually wanted, so I decided to let it pass. Must have been painful for him, don't you think? I mean, you take a certain action to get a reaction, but the reaction never comes.

That's how I deal with most haters. I walk away because I don't want to be dragged down to their level. I mean, what's the point in doing so? You waste precious energy if you give in to haters. So let it slide - be the bigger man! You only have to react when they keep on trying.

Those hateful comments that miss don't need a diss.

126. FREEDOM LEADS TO CREATIVITY.

I'm a very creative person; I need freedom to express myself. That's probably why I didn't excel in school or in restricted environments.

Always look for an environment that gives you a lot of freedom while you still have some rules to follow. There need to be rules, but they shouldn't restrict you too much. People never understand this, but it's hard to stand out if you have to perform in a restricted environment. Don't you feel better when you're able to be yourself?

There are gyms in Belgium who still force people to train with their left leg forward. Really stupid if you ask me, but that's the old school and some people want to keep it that way. Some people even do really good in those environments but I don't. So be aware of how what you need and change your environment if you have to.

127. WRITE AT NIGHT

I still believe that everybody should write and do martial arts. But we're going to talk about just the writing now.

You should try to write at night because that's probably a time when you're alone. I often do it 30-60 minutes before bed. I think about things during the day which upset me or turned out to be an obstacle, then I write about them. I just describe the events, how I felt and then I try to design some kind of resolution.

I do this with everything. I even do it when times are going great because you need to understand yourself in the good and the bad times.

So buy yourself a notebook and start writing. This only takes five minutes a day at a minimum. But you'll grow as a person and that's extremely important!

128. NEVER COMPARE YOUR TIMELINE TO SOMEONE ELSE'S

People like to compare themselves to others, but that's extremely dangerous.

I mean, I would be pretty depressed if I did something like that. I'm 25, live at home, don't own a car, I'm single, I don't have a degree, and so on.

People should realize that we all achieve things in life at different times. I know a woman that met the love of her life at 55. She could have cried about the fact that all her friends had kids and other things that she didn't have, but she didn't. She focused on herself and look at what happened.

The lesson here is to do everything at your own pace. There is no set date to achieve things; that's just society that wants you to believe something like that. You don't need to be married with a kid at 25 and you don't need to be divorced at 44 with a kid either. Go after what you really want, but do it at your own pace.

129. THE SECRET BEHIND MY MINDSET

People always wonder how it is that I never give up. Well, the reason is pretty damn simple: I overcame depression and suicidal tendencies. Now I have the feeling that I can overcome anything.

I'm not delusional, of course, but I mean that this was a pretty life-changing event that has shaped me in a good way. So what is your life changing event? Has there been a time in your life where you almost gave up but eventually got through?

If you've been there, great! Now you can use it to put things in perspective. Getting rejected might hurt, but it's not that bad if you compare it to being depressed. I mean, there are levels to feeling pain in life.

Some events in life might break us, and it's easy to feel sorry for ourselves, but that's not the solution. Remember that you had it worse and you overcame that as well. So tell me, why are you still complaining?!

130. A LIFE LESSON FROM A 92-YEAR-OLD.

A 92-year-old once said that life's short. I was pretty shocked when I heard this at first because that person had lived so much longer than me. But it's true: life is short, because we don't know when we're going to die and time flies by.

Life is short, but there are still people who do jobs that they don't like, stay in toxic marriages and so on. We all assume that we're going to live forever, but we won't . We're going to die one day, so it's better to live life to the fullest before the reaper visits us.

Could you die in peace knowing that you could have gotten more out of life? Could you live with the fact that you were together with someone who didn't respect you?

I can give tons of examples, but the main takeaway is simple. Life is short, so live accordingly. Just be smart if you live accordingly. Don't push it.

131. NEVER PRETEND YOU'RE OK

Every person has certain dreams. It's normal to have these, but most people claim that they're OK when they fail to achieve them.

Are you sure that you're OK? You still have time to achieve the things that you want. Why give up now? Michael Bisping was 37 when he won the world title in the UFC, a he fight he took on two weeks' notice. He had always come short of the championship before, but at 37 he got what he was working towards. I genuinely love this story because he Bisping was such a hardworking guy.

So don't lie to yourself. What do you really want? What are your dreams, goals and desires? Write them down and put a date on them, but never, ever pretend that you're OK with a life that you don't like. It's a like taking the highway to depression. It's reckless and dangerous.

132. YOU'RE ALWAYS "GOOD"!

I always tell people that I'm doing fine when they ask me how I'm doing. Some people are put off by this, but I do it for two simple reasons.

First of all, most people don't care about how you feel. Second of all, you give power to an event the moment you say you're sad because of it. You're still alive, right? Still breathing? Well, you're good then. There is no excuse for playing the victim and there is no excuse for complaining all the time.

Sometimes you need to realize how blessed you really are. The bad times are, in the end, the good times. People who're not able to see this have a giant problem because life is full of unpleasant surprises for them.

So how are you feeling right now?

Pretty good??

I thought so!

133. LEARN FROM OTHER PEOPLE'S MISTAKES

I always try to learn things from other people. But I mostly try to figure out what lessons their errors can offer me.

Donald "Cowboy" Cerrone recently said in an interview that he learned enjoy the walkout to the cage more then he used to. He let it all soak in and he really enjoyed the process. Similarly, my grandfather once said that he would have followed his dream if he hadn't listened to his environment.

Do you get where I'm going? Most people learn things in life and we all learn them at different paces. So why not pick other people's brain? Isn't that going to make you a lot stronger?

We can actually benefit from other people's mistakes. We can make sure that we don't make the same mistakes. That makes sure that we're a little bit ahead of the curve. It's better to learn a lesson from someone else than to learn a lesson when it's too late.

134. GO ALL-IN OR ALL-OUT

People mostly half-ass things. They want to fight in the UFC, but they only train three hours a week. It doesn't work like that. You really need to put a lot of time and energy into things when you are attempting something. You can't expect to be great if you barely put time into it.

I'll give you an example of my own life. I usually work on the blog for about six hours a week maximum, but I train 17 to 18 hours a week. Can you guess where my priorities are? Can you guess what I want in life? I decided to go all-in ,and then go-all out in one thing, and everything else is a distraction.

There are a lot of people who don't get this mindset, but they will only get it when they finally find something that they really like. That's the only thing that might help them realize this.

135. I'M NOT DISCIPLINED, I JUST LIKE WHAT I DO

I have zero discipline, because I won't do things that I don't like. Like going to college. still, people think that I'm super disciplined because I spend so much time in the gym.

The reality is that I just found something that I really liked. I was immediately hooked when I tried MMA. I became completely obsessed by it and I've never had something like that before. I was pretty lazy when I was younger. I would've never believed that I was going to become that intense.

So find something that you really like and spend a lot of time doing it. That's a way to be happy. People will think that you're obsessed, which is true to some degree, but the real secret is that you like what you're doing. Most people don't get this because they don't like what they're doing. That's why they don't see how you can spend so much time doing something. I train a lot a week, but I would never study a college course for the same amount of time a week.

136. PEOPLE WILL ALWAYS FIND AN EXCUSE (OTHERWISE THEY'LL GOOGLE ONE)

I've always wanted to share what I have learned since I started my self- development journey. I mean, wouldn't it be great if all people could become better?

I quickly realized that it was a pipe dream. Most of them didn't want to change or they can't keep up with the pace and will be left behind. In the end, people will always look for the easiest way. Even I'm prone to it from time to time, but I also realize that it's a case of easy come, easy go. It's just better to face the fact that you're either are going to put in the work and get better or be lazy and get bitter.

The strange thing is that some people sometimes put more effort into searching for an excuse than doing the work. Really weird, because doing the work will give you better results than constantly looking for excuses.

137. HARD WORK BEATS TALENT WHEN TALENT DOESN'T WORK HARD

Did you know that I was one of my classes' worst writers in high school and college? Did you also know that one of my teachers told me that I should never try sports because I wasn't made for them? But now we are in 2019. Now I'm training 17 hours a week while I've run my own blog for nearly three years now.

Crazy, right?

So what happened? Did a magical fairy visit me to sprinkle some talent dust over me? No, I just put in the work and got better over time. This goes for both blogging and MMA. I just trained so much when I started that it looked like I was a natural who picked things up quickly, but what people didn't see was that I was practicing for hours in my garden until I got the moves right.

Aside from that, I've noticed that people who pick up things easily usually don't put a lot of effort into things. They just figure that they'll be good at it over time and then they end up facing someone who's really good at it down the road. I suppose that I don't have to explain what happens then, right?

138. DON'T WORRY ABOUT THE FUTURE JUST WORK HARD

There are tons of people who worry about the future. Actually, they worry about others' future at the same time. It's useless to worry since this drains energy from you. This won't bring you happiness, just more negative thoughts and endless problems. Besides how many fears have become reality in your life? I can't remember a single one of my fears that has become reality, unless the monster under the bed suddenly shows up after all these years.

Fear lies to you. Fear dissuades you from trying to conquer it. After a while, you'll get out of this mindset and feel happiness. Work towards your goals and you'll notice that everything will work out for you. It just takes time and patience. Those are two things that most people neglect. Aside from that, they're just afraid of the unknown, but the unknown is what makes life so interesting.

139. I WILL NEVER PLAY THE LOTTERY.

People want to play the lottery because they want to be rich and escape their jobs. But do you really win if you win the lottery? You'll lose friends and family members because they're jealous. That doesn't sound like a win, does it? Aside from that, you'll become bored pretty quickly and you'll be broke in about five years. Then you'll have to return to your old job which you completely hated.

I don't know about you, but it all sounds so depressing to me. I don't want to return to my old job after I've left it behind. So I don't play the lottery because I know that it's a very dangerous gamble that'll not pay off in the long run. It could be the worst thing that ever happens to someone.

140. FAMILY IS A FANCY WORD

That there was a period in which I didn't talk to my brother. We didn't talk for two months and after that, we barely talked. In fact, we still don't talk a lot. The reason why is pretty simple: he can't engage in a proper conversation. He'll use profane language, often directed at me. I just got sick of it at one point. So I decided to let him be.

I have other family members to which I barely talk, as well. Most of them I ignore because they're hateful people who always want the worst for others. I don't want to talk to them because I don't want to be like them.

People always claim that family is everything but I disagree. Good family members are everything and good friends can be like family. Remember this. There are a lot of people who put up with bad behavior from family members and suffer as a result. Don't be like them. Cut the bad ones out and spend time with the good ones.

141. YOU'RE WIRED TO BE TIRED

A lot of people claim that they're tired all the time. This might be true, but are they really tired? I mean, how can you be tired if you never work out or do active things? It's because you're wired to be tired. You're just used to it. You're tired when you wake up, you're tired when you're awake, and so on.

My boss recently asked my where all my energy comes from. He didn't understand how it was that I was able to run in the morning and train at night. The reason is pretty damn simple. My body is trained to be active. My body feels great after training.

Of course I'm tired, but it's another kind of tired. It's not draining. It feels like I'm alive. The main takeaway here is that most people lead very sedentary lifestyles combined with unhealthy diets. Our bodies are not designed to be used like this. Be active, get outside. Run or lift, do martial arts... Do something, but don't sit on your ass all day. You'll gain nothing from it.

142. I LEARNED SOME VALUABLE LESSONS AFTER A SERIES OF INJURIES

There was a period of time in which I seemed to be having one injury after the other, all of which were my fault. I was focused on training, but I didn't focus on recovery, so I was injured all the time.

This string of injuries taught me that it's easy to feel sorry for myself. That's the easiest thing that you could do, but eventually I learned how to use those periods to my advantage. I improved my mindset a lot during these periods. Now I focus on mental health during my periods of injury because a bad mindset will lead to a sick body.

I also learned that you shouldn't take painkillers or all that other stuff. I used turmeric and other natural herbs during my injuries. Plus, I learned that you can still train. I had a knee injury, but that didn't mean that I couldn't train my upper body twice a week. Always try to remain active when you're injured if it's possible.

143. DO IT NOW INSTEAD OF TOMORROW AND YOU WON'T FEEL SORROW

Most people have claimed, at one point or another, that they'll start something tomorrow. They'll ask their dream girl to go on a date when tomorrow arrives. They'll start getting in shape as soon as tomorrow arrives. It's a dangerous mindset because tomorrow will come, but the chances that you'll take action are a lot smaller.

Many people have made the claim that it's the last day that they'll eat unhealthy food in front of the television. It's easy to be lazy. It's really the easiest thing in the whole world. You just have to do nothing but watch television all day. No wonder that so many people do this. There are so many distractions in life which most people can't resist. These distractions put people to sleep.

You should avoid these distractions since they'll make sure

that you get nothing more out of life. You should force your-self to get out of that precious comfort zone and take action no matter what.

144. FORGIVENESS IS A VERY POWERFUL TOOL

Remember the fact that my old trainer talked smack about me on social media? I forgave him. I don't forget, but I do forgive.

You see, holding grudges is the dumbest thing that you can do because you're carrying extra weight around. That extra weight will drag you down in the end. Some people will hurt you and some people will even do everything in their power to take you down. Still, you can never hold grudges. You have to be aware of the fact that they're the ones who're poisoning their selves, so don't stoop to their level. Lift yourself up, forgive and move on.

An easy way to remember this is that it's like running to the store with an empty backpack, then running back with your groceries. You'll quickly realize that it's harder to run with that extra weight, so don't do it. Don't keep on running with that extra weight. Throw it off and you'll be free. Just make sure that you don't throw your groceries away. That would be stupid.

145. RESPECT IS AN EXTREMELY THOUGHTFUL ACT

Ever heard of Mario Balotelli? He's an Italian striker who opted not to cheer when he scored twice. His team went to the finals and everyone was surprised. A reporter asked him why he didn't cheer and his response was pretty unusual. He told the man that he was just doing his job. He said that he had never seen a postman cheer when he posted a letter. It's a strange comparison that doesn't show much respect for the fans.

I had completely forgotten about this incident until I traveled to Spain. On the way home, there were some people who didn't clap when the pilot landed the plane. Some people assumed that it was reasonable not to clap because the pilot was just doing his his job. They neglected the fact that he had to land safely in order to protect more than 100 lives. Doesn't he deserve applause for the important job he performed?

146. CHOICES SHAPE YOUR LIFE WHETHER YOU LIKE IT OR NOT

The "butterfly effect" is a term used to describe these little choices. One little choice can change your whole life. It may sound stupid, but that's really how things go in life.

Most people won't work if they don't have to, but they all want a successful life. Why don't you try to aim for one successful hour per day? Those hours will multiply soon enough. One hour will turn into a day, a day will turn into a week, and you'll have a successful life before you even know it, all based on your own choices.

Do you get what I'm trying to say?

Your choices may seem small or insignificant in he moment, but they determine the outcome of your life. Your choices eventually become your lifestyle. I didn't believe this when I was younger, but I've seen the effect of it. Most people just slowly become lazier and more depressed because they're constantly making poor choices. They do it because that one little choice turns into a habit over time.

147. A FANCY DEGREE WILL NEVER IMPRESS ME

Some people like to show off their degree, or even multiple degrees. They'll come across as really smart, well, at least according to our society.

It's actually a bit funny that people need a piece of paper to prove that they're smart. And someone gives you this piece of paper while it's entirely possible that you've cheated to pass every test. So even though you've faked it all, the piece of paper proves to 99% of people that you are smart.

A bit weird, right? I mean, it does sounds a bit dumb, doesn't it?

People with a degree also have a higher change to be forgiven extremely quickly. Here's are a couple real life examples: "He's an alcoholic, but he has three degrees, so it's alright... She doesn't do shit with her life and constantly hurts people, but she's almost an engineer, so it's all fine."

People seem to be obsessed with that piece of paper and I don't get it, to be honest. There are multiple hidden traps here.

148. LOOK AT RESULTS, NOT AT RANKS

I'll never forget my first day in my old gym. My old trainer wanted to prove to me how good he really was. He low kicked the shit out of my leg (he really had a good low kick), then bragged about his black belt in MMA and his blue belt that he'd received from Robin Gracie.

It took me two years to figure out that he wasn't as well trained as he pretended to be. He pretended that he was good but wasn't.

My new trainer, on the other hand, never mentioned his achievements, even though he's a European kickboxing champ. But everybody knows how good he is. He doesn't have to showboat because he's widely known as one of the best trainers in Belgium.

Watch out for people who need external sources to prove how good they are. They're mostly not that good, but they like to delude themselves and others into believing that they are.

149. THE PROCESS IS A LOT MORE ADDICTIVE THAN THE END RESULT

The process is so addictive because it enables you to get better every single day. You really become better, but you just won't notice the improvements each and every day. All the small achievements add up after a while. That's what makes is so addictive and that's what most people neglect.

You see this a lot in sports. People get their pro status and have promising careers. But they never get the career that most people predicted they would have. That's because those people tended to focused on the end result instead of the process. It's the process that makes you better, not the end result.

That's why some people keep on practicing after training. They just want to get better while others just want to go home. You'll find me at the heavy end bag before and after training, otherwise you'll see me stretching. Most people get into the gym and treat it like a bar. They just want to talk to others, but you won't learn a lot from that. Focus on the process and aim for the end result. Not the other way around.

150. THE GENERATION THAT REJECTS RELATIONS LIVES IN FRUSTRATION

We're living in weird times these days. People are constantly on dating apps, but they don't want relationships. They want to share pictures with #couplegoals, but they don't want to put in the work to actually make the relationship work. It's something that I've seen for many years now. They all want friends with benefits, though. They all want the fun things that come with a relationship but without the commitment.

So are we really a weaker generation? I believe so, to be honest. What kind of person are you if you want all the good and not the bad? There's no balance that way. (I'm referring to yin and yang). You need the bad to appreciate the good. Besides, most people who're living the "fuck buddy" lifestyle deep down want a relationship, but somehow they ignore this and that's why they're so unhappy.

151. MENTAL HEALTH IS CRUCIAL IN LIFE

A lot of people neglect their mental health these days. They don't get that it's so important! They constantly pop pills and pay bills. It's an empty lifestyle because they don't see the hidden danger behind the pill-popping. Popping pills kills. I mean, you are the source of your own problems. You've got the wrong mindset and you're trying to solve it with pills. Do you really expect that this approach is going to work?

Let me break it to you gently: a lot of people become dumber and dumber as they age, but they don't understand why. I understand why and they don't like the answer. They don't read books, they only chase looks.

There are a lot of people who laugh at me when I tell them that I meditate, but it feels so damn good to do it. It empties my mind and relaxes me. Some will joke that only monks do it, but I don't care. "Mens sana in corpore sano" is a saying for a reason.

152. KARMA WILL CATCH UP WITH

YOU (AND YOU DESERVE IT)

Some people do a lot of bad stuff but always seem to get away with it. Others start to wonder how they do it, then inevitably start to envy them after a while. There's nothing to envy here. Those people are mostly bad and dark inside. They're dumb as fuck and they have big egos to boot.

It doesn't matter how long they get away with all their acts because the tides will change eventually. Suddenly, one day, they will get what they really deserve. Their whole act will be exposed and many onlookers won't be surprised about the outcome.

The people who do bad stuff can get into a comfort zone for sure. But can you guess what they'll do when adversity pays a visit? They'll act like a victim, claiming they don't deserve this. The universe tried to teach them a big lesson and they cried about it. Zero problems are solved in that way. We all do dumb things in life. Yes, I have done dumb things, too, but I have paid the price and learned my lesson.

153. A WIN OR A LOSS IN LIFE SHOULDN'T DEFINE WHO YOU ARE

People who win are winners and people who lose are losers, at least according to most people. But this isn't true, since some people become stronger after a loss. They come back as changed men and surprise everyone.

Most people can't handle a loss because it hurts their ego. How many of you have claimed that you didn't deserve some sort of treatment at one point in your life? That's ego-bound thinking. You don't deserve anything in life.

Really, Alex? Nothing?

Absolutely nothing. Your life was the only gift that you've ever received. The rest is up to you, but that's something that most people can't handle. Let's take a look at how you should handle every loss in life.

154. HOW TO HANDLE A LOSS LIKE A BOSS

Losing isn't tough, it's just a part of life. It stings, that's for sure, but everybody loses in life. However, most people just give up way too soon. Let me explain.

What do you do when you break a bowl? You clean it up and throw it away, right? Well, in Japan, they repair it with some kind of golden glue. It's called *Kintsugi*. It's to help remind them that the bowl is now stronger in the places that had been broken.

Most people break and never recover from it. You should celebrate all adversity. You should take it head on because you will become better at dealing with it in the future. There's no place for excuses. What doesn't kill you makes you stronger, so why would you make yourself weaker? Just carry on and learn.

155. BEING ON A WIN STREAK IS DANGEROUS

We like to win since the feeling is extremely addictive. We get a boost in powerful brain chemicals and completely lose control. We become so confident that we become overconfident after a while. We get into a comfort zone and that's when we suffer our most devastating losses.

It'll hurt without a doubt. You can't learn anything from a win, which is what most people don't seem to realize. They want to be winners, so they focus on the winners. Those people miss the point completely since they neglect all the losses from those people.

Don't be a fan boy. Be realistic. Everybody has wins and losses in life. Some just handle them a bit better than others.

156. FORGOT ABOUT A WIN OR A LOSS

So some people call themselves "winners" and others call themselves "losers" based on their respective experiences. It's all a matter of perception; you need to realize that. You aren't a winner or a loser. You're a human being on a journey.

You see, you just have to work your ass off. Give it your all and realize that you still win even if you lose. Some remember only the wins and losses, but you should focus on something completely different. Focus on the process, since it's so addicting. That's the only thing that you should ever remember.

I once wrote a blog post about what I had learned over the course of a year. In it, I never claimed that I won or lost anything. I just loved the whole process no matter what happened. Yes, even if life gave me some hardship, I loved it, since it's all part of life.

You win some and you lose some, but life goes on in the end.

157. TRAVELING IS THE MOST SUBTLE FORM OF ESCAPISM

E ver noticed that people have the tendency to blow a lot money when they travel? They throw away 1000s of dollars to enjoy a eight-day vacation at a luxury hotel while sitting at the pool all day. What a waste of money. These people are probably extremely unhappy. They travel to escape their job, which they hate. That's pretty sad, don't you agree? Because they eventually have to return to the job they hate after they've blown all their money. This process continues until they figure it out, get depressed or hit retirement.

You should never travel to escape your own problems. You'll just take them with you. Remember that, because it might save you a lot of money.

158. LEADING AN UNHAPPY LIFE WITH A NON- FUTURE WIFE

I knew a guy who once dated a girl and very quickly they decided to travel together. They didn't really know one another, but they guy really wanted to get laid. So they booked an extremely fancy trip and shared everything on Instagram. They looked very happy, but the truth came out pretty fast. The trip had been a complete nightmare and the guy was sad that he blew a lot of his money.

The lesson here is pretty simple: don't go overboard when you meet someone new. They could have stayed in Belgium and gotten to know one another locally. It would have cost a lot less money, but the end result would have been the same. They would have broken up anyways. Relationship aren't easy, so there's no need to make them harder.

159. DREAM KILLERS ARE EGOCENTRIC PEOPLE WITHOUT REALIZING IT

People always try to keep others down when they're about to chase their dreams. I once met a woman who had gotten an offer to move to the States for work. She would have gotten everything (house included), but she didn't go because of her mom. Her mom wanted her to stay in Belgium because she didn't want to go to the States.

The mom regretted her action and hoped that her daughter would get a second chance, but I highly doubt that this'll happen. These opportunities are pretty rare. You can never stand in someone else's way. It's extremely selfish. Support people when they're about to achieve their dreams. Be happy for them and never hold them down. It's really stupid to act that way. They'll remember it in the long run.

160. THERE'S SOMETHING WRONG WITH THE EDUCATION SYSTEM

The education system makes you hate learning. Did you hate to learn all that useful stuff as well? Did you hate reading because of all those book reports? I know that I did. I didn't see the point in learning stuff that you didn't need in real life. Most people hate learning and that's why they don't evolve any further. They get dumb and dumber without realizing it.

The education system doesn't reward the people who work hard. There are two kinds of students: the ones who work hard and the ones who party hard. In the end, they all get the same degree and the same paycheck. Why would you even bother working hard if the end results were just going to be the same?

This is something that I really hated about college. I need something that motivates me and this didn't motivate me at all. The lazy ones may be happy with their approach, but it's not really fair.

161. LOSERS FOCUS ON WINNERS, WINNERS FOCUS ON WINNING

You need to focus all your energy on winning if you want to be a winner. You need to be driven and aiming for the end goal. You need to perform in the zone because that's where you're at your best.

Can you guess what happens when you're constantly focusing on other people instead of yourself?

You'll drop out of the zone. This is one of the reasons why you lose. You weren't present in the moment; the moment caught up with you. You'll get a reality check as soon as you see someone else win.

This is also applicable for the process before competition or for life in general. You need to focus on what matters, not on how much you hate someone. You're wasting precious time. There are more important things in life that most people don't seem to want to pursue. They claim that every rich person got rich by breaking laws or stealing from others.

They neglect all the work that these people have put in. But I get why they think like this. Do you?

162. SMALL TALK IS BORING

Have you ever been in a conversation in which the participants didn't go beyond the small talk? There's a reason why these conversations are so damn boring and don't last that long. They address topics which are too obvious to talk about.

A lot of people like to talk about the weather, but everybody can see and feel that it's cold. It's really not a big deal. You just know that there's an awkward silence coming ahead when people start to talk about the weather.

I've noticed that a lot of normal people like to have small talk. These people try to talk with me, but the conversations don't last that long since they ask questions that can be answered with just a single word. I'm not going to talk about the upcoming weather. That's a waste of time and far from interesting.

Ask these questions to be more interesting. What do you want to do before you die? What would you do if you die tomorrow? What's the meaning of life according to you?

People who can't answer these question are probably people who use small talk all the time, and those people are bored all the time, as well. Use these questions to be more interesting.

163. EXCUSES WILL MAKE SURE THAT YOU'LL NEVER GROW

We are fond of making excuses these days. These excuses are a curse. People don't get this because they start to believe their own excuses over time. They'll start to act like a victim after a while because they are always affected by external things that block their progress.

The reality is that they're the ones who're blocking their potential. What's even worse is when you call them out on their behavior, to which to reply by defending their own excuses.

Rationalizing your excuses is one of the most dangerous things that you can do since you'll be stuck with your rationale. You'll never achieve a single thing if you've fallen into this habit. It's really all up to you. You've got a tremendous power in your hands and you're wasting it by making excuses all the time.

164. MY WAY IS A WAY, BUT IT'S NOT THE WAY (PART II)

A lot of people say things like: "it's my way or the high-way." This is probably one of the dumbest things that I've ever heard. What works for one person might not work for another. You can try to copy people all your life, but you'll just be a good copycat. I mean, how many cover bands have actually become more popular than the original? NONE!

This is something that I realized pretty soon after I started my self-development journey. I didn't want to be a cheap dupli-cate. I wanted to be an original. Give credit to the people who influenced you, but go your own way.

People have to realize that they've got a unique voice inside of them. There's really nothing more valuable than you. You are unique, you are special. There will never be someone just as you are. We all live life in different ways. We all have different experiences and different insight that are valuable to others.

165. ALWAYS BE EXTREMELY GRATEFUL

You can't be grateful and depressed simultaneously. It's literally impossible. Just try it. Most of you will still feel depressed since most of us are experts at sweating the small stuff. I once heard a person claim that it was impossible to be happy when the weather wasn't great. I'm guessing that that person wasn't pleasant to be around during winter.

You should become a cold warrior instead of a warm worrier. Stop sweating the small stuff; it's a waste of time. You'll never be able to appreciate the good if you can't accept the bad. You'll end up with a life full of problems that you can't control anymore. Your life will turn into a dramatic rollercoaster which ain't a fun ride.

166. PERCEPTION DEFINES YOUR REALITY

Perception is something that can make or break you. Perception can be your best friend or your worst enemy. Most people do not get this. Something happens in life upon which they're not able to reflect. They act like victims and, slowly but surely, get more and more depressed.

Life will feel like a living hell if you don't act upon your own life. Once again: perception can make or break you. I'll use my own life to show you what I mean. Most people assume that I'm someone special because I'm doing things that they can't. Well, they assume that they can't. They're also afraid to do it. Fear is what's holding them down, but that same fear is motivating me.

I'm not extraordinary. I'm just an ordinary guy who once was just an average Joe. You can do what I can do if you're willing to put in the time and the work. Most people don't really understand me when I say this, but we're all just human. It's all about perception. The glass can be either half full or half empty. There is no right or wrong answer to this question since the glass is always half full and half empty. That, my friends, is perception. It's realizing that there are always two ways of viewing things. You've got to choose the right perception if you want to enjoy life.

167. PRIDE SERVES THE EGO, BUT IT DOESN'T SERVE YOU

S ome people feel superior to others. It all has to do with pride.

Most people are proud that they've earned a degree; they instantly don't want to do a whole selection of jobs because they've got that degree. Your pride is killing you here. I mean, do you realize what you're saying? You're saying that you're better than another human being because you've got a piece of paper and they don't.

This mindset is sickening, in my opinion. Your degree doesn't matter. What matters is your mindset. Yes, I've done shit jobs, but I did them even when I was still in college. There wasn't a single moment when I felt better than the others. I was bored a lot, that's for sure, but I never placed myself above another person. That's vain and pretentious. You should be ashamed that you're thinking like this. A job is a job and all human beings are equal.

168. YOU DON'T SEE SKIN COLOR? ARE YOU FUCKING BLIND??

There are people who claim that they look beyond skin color, which is absurd if you ask me. I mean, it's pretty obvious that some people have a different skin color. This is mostly used by people who're extremely racist but don't want to admit it. So they put up an act.

"Bro, I don't judge people based on their skin color." I've heard this so many times. Makes me sick, to be honest. There are obvious differences, but you shouldn't judge people based upon them. I never quite understood why people judged others based on their race. A white asshole remains an asshole. Just think about that next time you hear someone make a stupid claim related to race.

We're all different, we should accept these differences and not judge people for them. I wholeheartedly thank you.

169. THE CRAVING FOR COMFORT IS A THREAT TO SOCIETY

The modern generation is just a bunch of couch potatoes. You shouldn't even be surprised since there are so many distractions these days. You can play video games all day, watch tons of television shows, and watch the whole *Star Wars* series again for the seventh time. Most people have just become social media zombies.

Being grateful doesn't even exist for those people. They're selfish, little twerps. They're walking around with big "like me" button strapped on their foreheads. Social media presents a fake image, so people start to judge their own lives based on fake facts. It's sad, but this is the modern-day reality.

Remember that the less you judge yourself and others, the happier you'll be. It's really that simple. Judging yourself and others reveals a weak mindset.

170. THE CRAVING FOR COMFORT AND GETTING INTO SHAPE

I remember that a guy asked me advice to get into shape. So I told him what he had to do, but I noticed that my answer didn't satisfy him.

"So you've got to work hard and eat right? That's not fair since professional athletes have their own chefs. That's why they're in great shape," he told me.

This is in the running for the "dumbest quote of the year" award, in my opinion. I don't have a personal chef, plus I know many people who are in great shape without having a personal chef.

People like this guy want to get food delivered to their tables, but they don't want to work to pay for it. You might not be surprised to know that he's even more out of shape now. He prefers to game and eat junk food instead of eating and sleeping right.

Choices shape your life whether you like it or not. He made a choice, now he's paying the price. Hard work pays off and this will never change. Stop hating on people who're getting or already are in a great shape.

171. WORK YOUR ASS OFF IN EVERYTHING YOU DO

Life is all about work ethic. It beats fear, according to Michael Jordan, and he was right. You need to work extremely hard in whatever you do. It doesn't matter that you've got a shit job. Just do your job and shut up. Nobody likes a crybaby or someone who acts like a victim.

I'm currently working in a garden center and I could do better things with my time, but I've got to work to make some money. I work my ass off without having regretted a single day. I'm in the prime of my life right now, so I'm going to make it count. You're going to die anyway, so it's better to act now instead of never. It doesn't matter where I am because I'll always work hard. There's no excuse for being lazy.

It's like my grandpa once said: "give it your all or don't do it at all."

172. ARE YOU DEAD OR ALIVE? THE ANSWER MIGHT SHOCK YOU!

There are two types of time according to Robert Greene. There's "dead time," in which people are passive and waiting. The opposite is "alive time." This is when people are active, acting, learning, and using every second that they've got.

You've got a choice on how you use your time and most people don't use it wisely. They don't realize that choices shape your life whether you like it or not. Those choices can make a huge difference in your life. People really neglect this. So you assume that you're alive, but you're not. You're lying to yourself and you know it. Stop pretending that you're OK - you're wasting precious time. Most people don't seem to get it because they lose their ability to think over time. That's one of the first things that I noticed after I had done multiple temporary jobs.

You can breathe, but that doesn't mean that you're alive.

173. YOU CAN'T OUTRUN FEAR, BUT CAN YOU CONQUER IT?

You know what you've got to be? Imaginative, strong-hearted. You must constantly try new things. Sometimes you'll win, sometimes you'll lose. But don't let anyone define your limits because of where you come from. Your only limit is your imagination.

It's all a matter of perception. You can simply because most people assume that they can't. Just go and live your dream. Remember this line: "you're stronger than you feel, smarter than you think, and braver than you believe." That's what it's all about.

Hard work is what it takes. Take your place in the circle of life. We're going to keep moving forward because nothing is impossible. Even miracles take a little time. Adventure is out there.

"If you can dream it, you can do it. Always remember that this whole thing started with a dream and a mouse." (Walt Disney)

174. A STORY ABOUT A BIKE RIDE

So I was riding my racing bike when I was passed by an elderly guy on an electric bike. I was like, "oh, hell no, you're not going to get ahead of me!"

I put in extra effort and passed the guy when I suddenly noticed some other people who were riding ahead of me. I passed them all on my way to visit my grandfather. I kept on pushing even when I faced a heavy headwind. I was showing what I was made of.

Then, I met another guy with a racing bike along the way, who I flew past, too. He put in some effort and eventually passed me. I saw a little smile on his face, but I knew that I would pass him again. I was riding a bit behind him when we came upon a steep bridge ahead of us. He was already on the bridge when I was hitting the beginning. So I took a deep breath and accelerated. I passed him while we were both climbing and heard him become frustrated. I never looked behind me. I never saw the guy again on the remaining part of the road. His spirit had broken.

175. THE BIKE ANALOGY THAT'LL CHANGE YOUR LIFE FOREVER

Did you see what I was getting with that story of my bike ride? It's pretty easy. You'll always have to put in the effort no matter what you do in life. It may be uncomfortable in the beginning, but you'll get the hang of it. You have to leave your comfort zone.

There will be a time where you suddenly aim towards a goal in life (in this case, it was my grandfather's house). You'll have to set little goals along the way to remain motivated (all the other people that were riding in front of me). And you know that you'll face some troubles along the way (the headwind).

Do you get it now? But what about the guy who passed me you ask? Well, in life, there will always people who pass you at a certain point. You'll be frustrated, but you are the one who controls how much time and effort you put in. So you just pass them eventually and move on.

A lot of people quit as soon as they have to do some extra

effort (the guy struggled on the bridge and was frustrated when I passed him). That part contains a valuable lesson, too. You can be the biggest or strongest guy in the whole world, but you'll never achieve anything if you lack the heart. Most people display a lack of heart. A lack of heart means that you'll never have a head start.

176. I'VE NEVER LOST A STREET FIGHT. HERE'S HOW I DO IT:

It's pretty damn simple: I just walk away. Skills have to pay bills, but they don't pay bills when I'm fighting someone in the street. Aside from that, it's extremely stupid and there are no rules. I've never been involved in a street fight and I don't intend to be.

Walking away turns you into the real winner of the fight.

"Hence to fight and conquer in all your battles is not supreme excellence; supreme excellence consists in breaking the enemy's resistance without fighting." (Sun Tzu)

177. NEVER GO THREE DAYS WITHOUT EXERCISE

Most people aren't consistent when it comes to working out. They just work out when they "feel like it." I don't always feel like it, but I do it anyway. A lot of sports have an off-season, but there's no off-season in MMA or other combat sports. You're only taking time off when you're injured. That's it - that's your time off. You go back in as soon as you're good to go again.

Usually, I'll return a bit sooner than later. I strongly believe you should never go three days without exercise. It's dangerous because you'll be able to make up excuses as to why you shouldn't work out. You're on the road to becoming out of shape once again. Can you guess when you'll get back on track? In Neveruary!

Those are the people who come up with terms like "good genetics" and other dumb stuff. It's hard work and dedication-. You won't get in shape by coming up with excuses. It's all about the grind.

178. FAIL FORWARD INSTEAD OF FALLING FORWARD

Some of us like to watch *The Walking Dead,* but in reality, they're just part of the walking dead themselves. They can't handle their own problems and they shell up as soon as they fail.

I've seen people cry just because they made a mistake. Every mistake is human, so it's better to accept that you made a mistake. You're going to make more mistakes in the future. Just accept it, learn your lesson and move on.

I recently witnessed a little kid learning to walk. It was the same thing over and over again. The kid got up, tried, fell down, cried, got back up, and tried again.

Why would you give up when you did something wrong? I mean, are you perfect in everything that you do? I don't think so. It's really something weird how some people behave in life. Fail forward. Don't be afraid to keep moving forward.

179. IT ALL STARTS WITH ONE. "ONE WHAT, ALEX?"

E verything starts with one simple action. My MMA journey was the result of me attending one training session.
The same goes for the blog: I uploaded one simple blog
and the momentum got going.

Most people don't seem to get this. They tend to overthink
everything and will just procrastinate until it's too late. Too
late to make the most out of it, which those people will regret.

So the message in this pretty simple: you have to take action
if you really want to do something. You have to take the first
step towards your goal and thinking about it won't help you
at all!

180. WHAT IS THE MEANING OF A DAY?

E very day is a test of your performance. You're given 24 hours and it's your task to make the most out of them.

I sleep eight hours these days. Sometimes I'll add an afternoon nap if I'm really tired, but that's only for 10 minutes. You've got 24 hours to make your day successful. You should succeed for yourself but also for the people who depend on you.

So in these 24 hours you can either work your ass off or binge your favorite show. You can rely on each hour passing, but you can't rely on what each hour will bring.

It could bring you failure. It could even bring you adversity. You can always start your day prepared so you don't have to waste a single second wondering what'll come. You face the challenges head on without a single hesitation. You get the job done and end every single day with the confidence that you can get up and do it all again tomorrow.

You've got 24 hours ahead of you. Will you make them count or will you sleep all your remaining time on this earth away? Snooze and you lose.

181. DO YOUR SURROUNDINGS REALLY MATTER IN LIFE?

So many people are fond of doing nothing, which they rationalize with dumb excuses. The truth is that your surroundings are a part of your life, but they shouldn't be allowed to keep you down. You should be grateful for the opportunity to prove them wrong.

"But Alex, my relationship is going downhill and I can't focus on anything!" Work on it or end it. Don't wait until things get better. Waiting is the worst things that you can do.

"But Alex, I really hate my job and I'm miserable all the time!" Quit and look for a better job.

Learn some new things while you've got more time in a day. You can learn new things just by reading. You can come up with excuses all day, but there's always a solution. Most people just don't want to take action because they're afraid. So they wait and wait and wait, claiming that they'll change everything when the time is right. I hate to break it to you, but

the time is never right. The odds will never be in your favor.
JUST DO IT.

182. CHANGE WILL NEVER HAPPEN OVERNIGHT

I know a lot of people think about improving themselves. They want to go on a diet, live healthier, be more active, read more, and so on.

This is all fine and good, but most people never get around to it and that's not fine. They somehow think that the change will happen overnight if they put in effort for some time. It just doesn't work like that.

You need to put in effort every single day. That's it. There's no magical fairy that'll make the change happen overnight. So stop chasing pipe dreams and get after it.

183. A REMARKABLE QUOTE BY A NARCISSIST.

Somebody once asked me if I had any advice on how to become a better person. So I said, "focus on yourself." Just after I said that, someone else wanted to be the smart guy and claimed that it was a narcissist trait to focus on yourself. The problem was that this guy was so full of himself but had never bettered himself. He was basically a narcissist, but he didn't see it.

I asked him, "how can you ever improve yourself if you never focus on yourself?" I mean, that's pretty impossible, right? You can't say "yes" to everybody and expect to become a better person.

I'm glad that I wasn't stuck in this mindset for a long period of time. I've heard multiple people who recovered from depression say that they became more selfish. I can vouch for this. You have to be selfish to be happy and reach your goals. You can't say no to people if you're not selfish. Forget what society tells you. You have to be selfish to make it.

184. MEETING WITH THE FAMILY GONE WRONG

My grandma once had a tenant who had had an interesting life. She never paid the rent on time but always traveled. Eventually, my niece googled her name and it turned that she had been involved in a reality show back in the day. She even found her Instagram, filled with pictures of her in bikinis.

My family obssessed over this woman. She was a topic at most family meetings. Once, they asked my opinion on it because I hadn't been very vocal about it. I said that I absolutely didn't care and that they all needed a hobby. The weird part was that they didn't see how their behavior was so toxic. They were hating on another person while they were enjoying cake and coffee.

This doesn't sound like a perfect, cozy Sunday if you ask me. I hated it, but I got a lot of hate thrown at me for telling them to use their time more wisely.

185. THE TRUTH HURTS...

In the last chapter, I talked about the time that I told some family members that they should get a hobby, after which they all got mad at me. It was a disgrace, according to my parents, and I got a lot of shit for it.

Why where they all so mad? Because I had struck a weak spot. They all knew that they were wasting time, but they were so caught up in the moment gossiping that they didn't see this coming. They all assumed that I would agree with them, but instead I told the truth. I basically did what nobody dared to do because of the social pressure.

Were they really mad because they heard that they needed to find a hobby? No. I just told them that they should invest their time a lot better because they're going to die one day. I'm pretty sure that they got it. People older than 50 often reflect on their mortality because their bodies are slowly falling apart.

The truth hurts, but it remains the truth.

186. THE TRUTH DOESN'T HURT ME

This is where it gets interesting, isn't it? Why would the truth hurt others but not me?

Well, the answer is pretty damn simple. I reflect a lot on my own behavior, so I mostly figure out stuff that I have to work on before other people see it. I have already corrected it or am correcting it by the time people point it out. So this means that it can't hurt me because I've already accepted it.

But what if they point out something that I haven't found out yet? Well, then I accept it and work on it. That's how I've improved so quickly as a martial artist. I'm always looking for immediate feedback to make me better. That's because I know that the only way to improve is to ask my coach feedback.

Same goes for life. The only way to improve is to accept your flaws and work on them. People spot those a lot easier than you, especially in the beginning. Learn to be ahead of the game and nobody will be able to upset you.

187. AGE DOESN'T DEFINE WISDOM

Some people assume that older people are always wiser, but is that really the case?

I know a guy who's 50. He always looks down on people who don't have a degree. He rarely gives out any advice or guidance on life. The reason why is simple. You can't gain wisdom if you've never lived life. It's like the guy who watches tons of MMA videos online. Sure, you can watch them all, but that doesn't make you a fighter.

It's easy to spot smart, older people. They're mostly joyful and they'll share their wisdom. Dumb, older people will force their "wisdom" on you.

Why would you follow the advice of an unhappy person? To be unhappy yourself? What's the point in doing so? A moron remains a moron when that person is older. Now he is just an old moron.

188. DEGREES DON'T MEASURE INTELLIGENCE, EITHER

Degrees are an ego thing to me. It's proof that even dumb people can be labeled as smart.

I'll never forget my last semester in college. We had a final on economics. I really understood the course; I was so proud of myself. Thirty minutes before the final started, a girl started asking me questions. She didn't understand anything, but she had mesmerized the all of her notes. Guess who passed with a high score and guess who almost didn't succeed at all? Me.

I didn't get a high score because that final was full of questions that checked if you could repeat what was in the course. You didn't have to understand it at all. I was so pissed when I saw this final. I dropped out not long after because I realized that you didn't need to be smart to be a parrot. Also, I noticed that "smart people" make poor life choices. But go to college or university if you want to do a job that requires a degree (like a doctor). Just take a good look at whom you surround yourself with.

189. WORRY AND YOU'LL DIE IN A HURRY

Ever seen people who worry a lot? Have you seen them after a while? They don't look so healthy, do they?

That's because those people mostly neglect their own health while they're so busy worrying. They mostly lack quality sleep because they're up all night worrying. They eat unhealthy food to kill the stress, or maybe they don't eat at all and instead fill their head with negative thoughts. So these people age a lot quicker and they die a lot sooner.

People who worry that they'll die young mostly die young anyway. Really sad but true. Other are so distracted by their worries that they die in a car accident or get hit by a car. Stop worrying and pay attention.

190. I'M NOT A ROLE MODEL

People started to contact me as my blog got more eyes on it. A few people even called me a "role model."

This was pretty crazy to a 24-year-old(at the time). I didn't see myself as a role model and I still don't see myself as one right now. I'd prefer to call myself a "real model" because I know that I've done and will still do a lot of things wrong. That's what's significant about growth. You fuck up, you learn and you move on. It would be stupid to deny this. The whole reason why my blog's so popular is because I admit these flaws and reflect on them. People seem to be drawn to this kind of honesty. So I'm not a role model. I'm a real model and I'm proud of it.

I use everything that's happened to me in the past to help others and myself. I lost everything at the age of 21. Now I'm on a path to regain everything back and gain even more. The cure in the pain is in the pain, remember?

191. NO LEVERAGE, NO DEAL.

There once was a guy who contacted me on Instagram. He really wanted to be on my podcast. I was pretty curious as to why he wanted to be on my podcast. So I asked him to explain why he should be on my podcast. He gave me multiple reasons but none that I could resonate with. I mean, you can try to sell yourself all you want, but trying to build your name off mine won't work. You have to give me a reason why I would invest my time in you. Both parties need to be able to win in this case.

The guy didn't have a blog, a podcast, a YouTube channel - nothing. I'm sure he wanted to start one, but that's not the point. I eventually agreed to let him on but only if he asked me questions. He agreed but didn't show up online at the scheduled time. He did this twice. He gave me a lame excuse why he didn't show up the first time. I didn't even bother asking the second time. The guy was a waste of time, so I don't contact him anymore.

192. THE UNWISE WATCH THE SAME THING TWICE

This was a reference to how most people live their lives. I got mocked a lot by people when I dropped out of college. But those people were all curious about how I spent my time since I was unemployed. Still, they all realized that I was up to something. They all claimed that they wouldn't be able to get up early and start their day.

So after a while, I asked them how they spend their time after they finished work. I got curious because I couldn't imagine what they were doing. Turns out that they were watching the same shows and movies over and over again. I couldn't wrap my head around it, to be honest. I still can't

They claimed to be wise, but do the wise watch the same thing twice? Or more than twice? I don't think so!

193. YOU CAN BE THE G.O.A.T. IF...

People always assume that you're the GOAT if you're the best in some kind of specialty, but that's not true. You can be the greatest of all time in everything you do.

You don't need fame and recognition to be a GOAT I once saw two young people with their little kid. They really enjoyed spending time with their son. Those people are both GOAT to me. I once heard a shop owner talk passionately about cheese and I was really interested. He's a GOAT to me.

Are you starting to get it? The GOAT is just a made-up term in our society. You're the GOAT if you're the best at what you do. So you can be the best parent, nurse, teacher, son, and so on without ever being on television. But does it really matter? I don't think so. You have to love the process and not everybody can push themselves to go through grueling workouts week after week. I believe you're the GOAT if you love the process.

194. YOU CAN DANCE OR GO INTO A TRANCE, BUT ESCAPING YOUR JOB? NOT A CHANCE!

Ever seen how most people lead their lives? They work the whole week, 9 to 5 every day, and then they go out on Friday and Saturday nights. It's something that they keep on doing for a long time. The weird part is that these types of people all want to escape their jobs, but claim that they can't.

Here's the thing: you can, but not with the lifestyle that you've got right now. You can't expect to get out of your job if you don't put in the work. That's just impossible.

This lifestyle puts you to sleep, so wake up before it's too late.

195. STUDY SUCCESS TO BE SUCCESSFUL

How can you be successful? That's a difficult question to answer, right? I mean, who doesn't want to live a successful life? We all do, don't we? And we all do it in our own way.

But how do we become successful? By studying success, of course? I've read one biography so far, but I've got two more that I'm planning to read. I've watched tons of interviews with people who talk about their rises to the top. Then I just find what suits me and my personality and go to work with it.

"The Notorious" Conor McGregor was on welfare before becoming a multi-millionaire and superstar success; other fighters commonly hold down normal jobs while trying to attain success. The journey to the destination doesn't matter. What matters is that you get there. Oh, and don't forget to enjoy the journey, otherwise you're screwed.

196. BAD TIMES DISAPPEAR, REAL MEN DON'T

This is a saying that's been used by a lot of wrestlers because wrestling is a grueling sport. Those guys are mostly extremely tough; they know that the bad times never last. They just keep on grinding until the good times come again.

It's like the weather. People always complain when it rains, but there's always sunshine after the rain. (Well, except here in Belgium.) So remember this when you're facing tough times again. They're just temporary events. They'll go away. So make sure that you don't go away because you'll regret it.

197. EVERYBODY SHOULD FIGHT, RIGHT??

I think that everybody should fight at least once in his life. I don't mean a street fight; I mean a fight with rules. You can pick the specific sport, but do a combat sport.

Now some people don't get why I keep on saying this, but the reason is pretty simple. We've all wondered what we're made off; sometimes we even make bold claims without knowing how to back them up. You can't make bold claims when you're being punched in the face. There's just no better way to test your mental toughness. You either grind and win or lose and need to get over it. It's a meaningful experience nonetheless. You might even like it and continue doing it! So why not give it a shot?

198. THE ONLY WAY TO BUILD A MEANINGFUL RELATIONSHIP.

People are always looking for "the one," so they look for a person who will support them. I've dated girls that have supported me, but it never works out. They couldn't handle the fact that I had so much stuff to do, so they bailed out.

The first thing that you need is a person that understands you because you're screwed if they don't understand. This'll lead to a lot of dumb arguments that require all your precious energy which should be invested in your projects/goals/dreams instead.

So what's the next step? Wel,l I would say either build an empire or make sure that you've both have stuff to do during the day. People who have no clue on how to spend their time are the worst to date when you're ambitious.

199. HATERS, HATERS EVERYWHERE

I wasn't very vocal about my blog when I started it, but the word got out eventually, of course. So suddenly my aunt and parents found out about my blog. They all hated on it and mocked me. My aunt even claimed that my life story was one of the dumbest things that she has ever read.

I didn't expected this, to be honest, and a lot of so-called "friends" did this to me, too. It pissed me off at first, but then I realized that these people just don't know any better. That was their attitude and I just needed to accept it. In fact, I've seen their attitudes change towards people they've hated in the past. You know what changed? Those people got more and more successful, and the haters sensed an increase in that wealth. So of course they suddenly supported those people. They changed for money. Isn't that funny?

200. ONLY DEAD FISH FOLLOW THE FLOW.

I told my osteopath about the fact that my family members and some "friends" had hated on my blog. The sad part was they didn't know even recognize all my goals. They hated it anyway because they had nothing better to do. My osteopath listened to my story and then he told me that I was on the right path. He said, "you know, only dead fish follow the flow."

He's right, you know. Why would you do what everybody else is doing? You'd only do that if your dreams were dead. I don't see any other reason why you should even consider following the masses. They don't even have a clue what they're doing. I mean, who are they following? Has anyone even thought about this? I prefer to swim, even if it means to swim against the current. Try to do the same. You'll like it once you've lived this life.

201. NO NORMS NOR VALUES

Some people just don't have norms and values, which this story will illustrate perfectly.

I was working temporarily at a meat factory and the boss was a real asshole. He was fake as fuck. So at lunch, people were complaining about the way he was behaving. They stopped the moment he came in. It was his birthday and he decided to treat everybody to some ice cream. So most of them accepted the treat, even though he gave it close to the time that we had to work again. They were all claiming that he was the greatest boss ever.

Guess what happened? Nobody returned to work on time, so he came furious into the cafeteria, telling everybody to get to work as soon as possible. Naturally, people started to complain again about him. He went from bad boss to good boss to bad boss again. Sad, right? People's opinions changed by ice cream.

202. WE'RE THE CRAZIES, BUT ARE WE REALLY?

This was something that my mentor, Sean "Muay Thai Guy" Fagan, told me. He told me this after we talked about the fact that some people hate on you. We are the crazies, according to 99% of the people, because we don't live like them (even though we have no desire to live like them).

Here's the joke about this whole thing: I think most people are crazy. I don't understand how they live to go out on Friday and sleep all weekend. I don't get why they want to work in a cubical until they're 65. I can't wrap my head around the fact that they really assume that they're going to enjoy retirement.

Those people are really crazy to me. But that's just the perspective issue, I guess. In the end, you've got to do what really makes you happy. But then the million-dollar question arises, of course: are they really happy??

203. BACK TO THE FUTURE.

Did you know that I used to be like most people back in the day? I always slept late, hated on other people, always lived for the weekend, and so on. I've turned my life around. And you know what's funny? I can't even recall living like I used to live. I don't even see why I liked it, to be honest. I'm like, "why did I live like that when it wasn't even enjoyable?" It was because I just didn't know any better.

You can only live your life like all the people around you. I just did what others did. And you know what? They now want to do what I do because they see how happy and energetic I am. Well, some of them to, anyway. The others just call me crazy.

204. GUYS WHO ONLY WANT HIGH TESTOSTERONE MISS THE POINT

The whole point of this blog was to teach guys how to increase their testosterone. I did this until I realized that it was a pipe dream. Guys want to be confident and they assume that it's directly related to having higher testosterone. But what's the point of that higher number if you don't use that confidence?

I know a guy who wanted to beat my testosterone count. So he took steroids, though there was something really odd about it. His numbers were fairly high, but he wasn't confident. It was just an act. He would explode when someone told him that he wasn't confident. He would defend himself and explain why he was actually so confident. It was painful to watch but a learning experience as well. I quickly realized that it's just a number. You just can't inject confidence. You have to work to be confident.

205. BIGGER, BETTER, STRONGER?

We live in a pretty vain society these days. Human beings are attracted to beautiful things - no doubt about it - but the rise of social media has even made it worse. So many guys want to become as big as possible just to bang as many girls as possible. Or they do it just out of insecurity.

Do you really think that you'll solve all your insecurity issues by getting bigger? Sure, you're big, but then what? You just turned yourself into the average meathead and you don't even realize it. So bigger, better, stronger? I don't think so. You're just bigger and stronger when it comes to looks and lifting weights. You're completely weak when it's mindset-related. People can spot this from a mile away.

206. THE EX-FILES: ARE YOU DOOMED?

So many people have had a ton of bad relationships and bad break- ups. It's like they're doomed. In fact, they often claim that they're doomed themselves, but is this really the case?Maybe they didn't learn anything from their previous relationship and that's why they made the same mistakes again.

I once knew a guy who had just gotten out of a relationship. Somehow he managed to score a date with a new girl pretty quickly. He was all over her, while she claimed that he was "the one." He was so convinced that he eagerly convinced me to meet her. So I agreed, but it only took me five minutes to tell that she was just the same, just like his ex-girlfriend. Same type of girl, same issues - just a different person.

She turned out to be not the one, which didn't surprise me. He blamed her for everything. Can you guess what happened when he scored a new date on Tinder? I'm sure you can. Same story all over again.

207. CHARACTER IS FATE, SO TAKE THE BAIT

Your character determines your fate. People with a strong character mostly have it better when it comes to the future. But people with weak characters have a stormy future ahead of them. They'll expose that weak character every time they're in a stressful situation. They break out of character, which leads smart people to quickly realize what kind of person they're dealing with.

So why take the bait, you ask? Well, women really like to test men. They test us all the time and they know they do it. Women are always looking for the guy that'll provide them with the best offspring. So why don't you see if you're really confident. Let a woman you date push your buttons and see how confident you really are. They'll walk all over you as soon as they see the chance. It happened to me in the past. I've seen it happen over and over again to other guys.

Machiavelli once claimed that fortune is like a woman. So how do you expect to have a great future if you can't even pass a test from a woman?

208. ACTIONS DETERMINE CHARACTER

You can't fake character when you're put on the spot. You need to be build that strong character. Nobody is born with it.

So how do I build up my character? By taking strong action. You'll always take strong actions when you're put on the spot. The reason why is simple: you are what you repeatedly do, so people who take weak actions have a weak character.

You can't turn this around overnight, although you might want to try. Strong actions are mostly the right actions. Sometimes this might be hard, but nobody claimed that it was going to be easy. Who wants an easy life anyways? That's just a sign of a weak character. So start to do the right thing and not the easy thing. Just watch how much you and your future improve by doing so. I challenge you!

209. THE DEATH OF INSTAGRAM MODELS

Every girl wants to be an Instagram model these days. This is a weird phenomenon, but I recently realized why 99% of Instagram models exist in the first place. It's because most men don't realize how valuable their time is.

Most of these Instagram models are beautiful, but they have nothing to offer. They're the female version of a meathead, but guys give them all their attention anyway. What would happen if men realized the value of their time? Well, most Instagram models would disappear like snow in the sun. That's a fact because their accounts wouldn't generate enough likes to keep afloat.

I knew a girl who wanted to be an Instagram model. But what really struck me was that all these accounts were the same and that tons of guys would slide into their DMs. Really crazy. Men, or people in general who realize that their time is valuable won't follow a lot of Instagram models. They know better.

210. HUMANS CAN OUTRUN A HORSE, SO WHY DO YOU PREFER TO SIT ON YOUR COUCH?

Did you know that humans can outrun a horse? A horse is faster, of course, but we can run a lot longer. This somehow explains how people were able to catch horses way back in the day. But that's not the point. The point is that our bodies are capable of doing a lot of work.

Your body is basically a machine and you're putting it into sleep mode by hanging out on the couch all day. I mean, why would you sit around all day if you're designed to be active? Stop being so damn lazy and start using your body! I don't ask you to run marathons or even run in general. I just ask you to be more active for the sake of your own health. Allow the machine to do what it was made to do.

211. HE SMILES ALL THE TIME, HE'S DELUSIONAL!

Someone once claimed that I had to be delusional because I smiled so much.

I don't think that makes me delusional. I've been through a lot, but I've survived it all so far and I realize now the beauty of life. That's why I smile. Sure, I face negative thoughts from time to time, but I'm aware that they're just temporary and that I can overcome them.

The same goes for you. Don't be deceived by your mind. Sometimes negative thoughts or self-doubt will pop up. Don't ignore them! Deal with what's at hand. The longer you wait to kill the monster, the bigger it gets. So face those thoughts right away and you'll be able to smile a lot more.

212. A SIMPLE CURE THAT SOLVES ALL YOUR WORRIES

Can you guess what all chronic worriers have in common? They have an abundance of time and no clue how to use it. People who worry a lot are mostly people who also do not take strong actions. However, time plays a giant factor as well.

I once heard a story about someone's grandma. She had worried about something for three days in a row. I didn't quite understand this, to be honest. This wouldn't be possible if she knew how to use her time wisely.

I have noticed that a lot of old people tend to be chronic worriers just because they have so much time to do so. But young people do this as well, particularly during the weekend, or at least I used to. There's a reason why so many people sit in front of television all day. So learn how to use your time more wisely and you won't have time to worry.

213. "IS SHE RICH?"

This was the first question that my grandma asked me when I started dating my former longtime girlfriend. "Is she rich?"

I didn't get it back then and I still don't get it to this day on. I mean, who cares about that? Wouldn't it be more important that she's a classy girl? This question is so stupid. What does it matter if someone is rich or not? Rich people have a larger amount of money than others, but that's about it. There are good and bad rich people, just like there are good and bad poor people.

Do you get where I'm going with this? This is one of the dumbest questions that I've ever heard! She still asks this question to this day. I mean, what if I had ended up with a rich girl who was a total bitch? Would that have been OK? The answer is probably yes, since my grandmother only talks about the ex of my nephew (a nice, rich girl). Her parents had a castle, you know. She'll be missed, I guess. But is she the one who's missed or just the money?

214. THE ONE QUESTION THAT YOU SHOULD ASK YOURSELF EVERY SINGLE DAY

There's one question that you should ask yourself every single day. The question is this:

"Am I really happy?"

This is hard to answer truthfully, especially in the beginning since you're prone to saying "yes" rather quickly. I mean, who in the world would admit that they're unhappy?

So many people just want to delude themselves, but answering this question might actually help you to get more out of life. This question is a way to find out what really makes you happy, because happiness is a pretty intense feeling, though sadness is intense as well. So ask this question every single day. You'll soon get to know yourself really well and you know what they say, right? "Self-knowledge is a way to wisdom."

215. I'M NOT FOR SALE, SO PLEASE FUCK OFF (PART I)

A lot of people stay in contact with certain family members to make sure that they get a piece of the pie when these people pass away. Being rich attracts a lot of fun people. They just pass time with you in order to get at your money.

I personally would never do it. I don't understand this mind-set at all. You're selling your self-worth and you don't even know that you'll get some money for certain. I wouldn't even do it if I knew that they would give me their money. I'm not going to live a life like that. Goddamn, it must be empty. I've seen family members do this. They even encouraged me to do it. So I was polite and told them, "please fuck off". I said "please," so that's pretty polite, right?

216. I'M NOT FOR SALE, SO PLEASE FUCK OFF (PART II)

O nce, a guy and I were practically best friends until I turned my life around. I suddenly realized how he had always looked down on me and still tried to do it. We eventually stopped talking, but he was still a part of the group of friends that I hung out with, which complicated things.

My group of friends met on a Friday and he was there as well. He needed as many people as necessary to help his father-in-law with a job. He played the part of the popular, perfect son-in-law, claiming that he knew a lot of people. He started asking around for help and finally came to me when everybody else had declined. He was desperate and said that they paid really well. I still declined. I seriously didn't care about the money and I can do a lot of better things than spending time with a guy who mostly talks smack behind my back.

217. WHY NORMAL JOBS ARE A JOKE

Normal jobs are here to keep you occupied. There, I said it.

I've never had a normal job where I was required to work eight hours in a row. It's stupid and people who really think that they're working eight hours in a row are delusional. I mean, just listen to a regular conversation between people who've done a job for a long time. First, they'll claim that they work barely at their job, which is a fact, and then they'll say, "but today I had to work really hard." I wonder if management moved the coffee machine so that they had to walk a little farther.

I noticed this rather quickly, so can you guess what I did when I was at my job? I finished work as soon as possible just to be able to study as much MMA-related stuff as possible. I'm not going to pretend that I'm busy like most people. That's the "take a broom" mentality. I don't like that and you shouldn't either if you're smart.

218. LOSING A BAD BOSS IS NO LOSS

I worked in a garden center where the boss had a weak character. She could be very manipulative. She would be nice when she needed to, but she would insult you when she was under pressure.

She got away with this behavior with every single employee for years but not with me. She insulted me once and I showed her that I didn't like it. Later that day, she asked me if I still liked working there. So I told her that I could quit whenever I wanted because I had weekly contracts back then. She stopped disrespecting me for a while, but then she did it again once I signed my fixed contract. That was a pretty bad move from her since that triggered me to write this book. She was still friendly most of the time and let me get away with a lot (stuff like getting in late), but I was determined to get out and she knew it. She just wouldn't accept it when the time was there.

219. SOLID ADVICE TO SAVE MONEY

People always claim that they're short on money. There's a reason why that's the case, of course. Stop buying stuff that you don't need!

I have one simple rule when it comes to spending money: I go check out the thing that I want and then I wait for 72 hours. I only buy it if I still think that I want it.

I've quickly come to realize that it's easy to spend money on things that we don't need. People see stuff as a source of happiness, but the only way to maintain that happiness is by buying new stuff all the time. The pattern goes as follows:

First, you buy something and you value it, so you're happy. Then the thing loses value over time, so you're less happy. The only thing that'll make you value it again is when you're about to lose it. That's when you're going to like it again. The point is this: don't buy stuff that you don't need. It's a giant waste of money.

220. THE FUNNY THING ABOUT... DISCOUNTS

I once worked for a guy who owned multiple supplement brands. He was wealthy and I could buy any of his supplements with a 40% discount as long as I worked there.

That got me wondering. How can he still make money while giving his employees such a big discount? I decided to ask him because I was really curious. He told me that the discount didn't matter; he still turned a profit. This surprised me, to be honest. He was a clever guy and gave out a lot of discounts to customers (mostly around 10%).

You know why? Because he knew that his customers would try to negotiate the price. So the sales prices was 10% higher than the amount of money that he actually wanted to collect. People who shopped at his store acted like a winner when they left the store. But the real winner was smiling right behind his desk.

221. THE FUNNY THING ABOUT... BRANDS

Remember that my former boss owned multiple supplement brands? He dialed it down to two in the end, all of which were fabricated in the same facility. They even had the same range of products. The one was just was a lot more expensive than the other. Guess which one sold the best? That's right, the one that was more expensive.

People who bought the more expensive brand were always claiming that it was so much better than the other brand. It made me laugh from time to time. They really believed this just because it was more expensive. There was practically zero difference between the products.

I learned a lot from my former boss, even more than I actually realized at the time. He was by far the best boss that I've ever had. This might sound weird coming from a guy who really hates normal jobs, but I mean it. I think it's even safe to say that I could've learned a lot more from him.

222. I DON'T BRAG WITH A GUCCI BAG

The last lesson goes for clothes as well. Brands are cheap if you buy them directly from the factory. I learned this from a girl who worked in a clothing store. A pair of pants was usually around 20 euros, but the price could go up to 200 when sold, depending on the brand.

Nowadays, a lot of people buy brands to prove that they're wealthy, or that's what they want you to believe, at least. Yet most rich people don't wear brands. Why is that? It's because they know the real value of money and will probably get paid to wear a certain brand.

So here's the joke: you're paying way too much money for brands purely in order to show off to other people. In reality, you're also paying a company to be a walking billboard. You know that you're paying to do this, right? Get it? I hope you do. Otherwise you're going to be broke in no time.

223. ALL THE INSTATRAVEL WILL UNRAVEL

There are a lot of Instagram posters that travel around the world, sharing their adventures along the way. It seems like they're living the dream, but don't let this fool you. One of the most popular travel accounts had to stop because the girl was in serious debt due to all the traveling.

You only see about 10% of people's lives on Instagram if you're lucky. You don't know these people, so don't worship them based on some happy pictures. I mean, would you be happy with a giant following while your debt keeps on increasing? Would you still envy that person if you knew that they're going to a bank to get a loan to "live the dream"? That's not a dream. It's a straight-up nightmare that was hidden from the public.

It's easy to put up an act on social media, but the truth will always come out.

224. ACHIEVE ALL YOUR DREAMS

What would happen if you didn't achieve your dreams? Nothing, right? You might be sad about it, but that would be it, wouldn't it? Not quite.

I've met a lot of people with broken dreams and they all have one thing in common: they all tried to force their kids to follow the dream that they had. Now these kids are suddenly chasing someone else's dream. The kids might achieve that dream, but I wonder who'll be the emptiest of the two.

It's really weird to try to relive all your broken dreams through your child. Why don't you make sure that you achieve your own dreams or at least try to achieve them? You might assume that not reaching your goals might be not that bad, but it really is. You might even undermine the happiness of your own kid(s). Don't do that to them.

225. WANT TO LIVE TOGETHER? DO THIS.

Couples who move in together usually have a phase where they fight all the time.

Why does this happen? It's because they stop chasing goals, seeing friends, going to the gym, and so on. They basically spend all their time together, which I understand because it's new and fun at first, but they'll be sick of one amother pretty quickly.

The only way to make it work is to actually make sure that you still do stuff outside of spending time with one another. Don't get too comfortable or you might break up and turn into a desperate "Tinderella" again. Sounds pretty horrible, doesn't it? I assumed that you would agree. So spend time together, but spend time without each other as well.

226. I WILL NEVER MAKE ANOTHER PERSON HAPPY

I will never make another person happy. I might add some happiness to their life, but I'll never be the source of their happiness. That's just impossible.

People who believe that you should make another person happy are delusional. You should make yourself happy and the other person should do the same. That's the only way that you can actually be happy together. It's weird that I have to explain this to people because they forget one simple thing. Can't the source of your happiness also be the source of your unhappiness? How would that work out when someone else gives you pain and joy without you being able to control it? Doesn't sound like a great plan. Yeah, I'd skip on that one.

227. I HAVE DREAMS, BUT NIGHTMARES TOO

We as people tend to become a little too confident when things are going well. We get caught up in the emotions and assume that we're kings of the world.

This all turns into a lot of pain when things go south. I once got rejected an hour before a second date. It's that event that led me to this lesson. I assumed that everything was going great until they suddenly weren't. So now I envision the good and the bad when I do things. Now I can live with the fact that I would get rejected an hour before a date. I can live with it because I've already seen it before.

You should try to do the same. The reason why is pretty simple: you can't be caught off-guard when you've seen it all.

228. YOU'RE NOT MADE TO BE "SINGLE AND READY TO MINGLE"

I call this the "happy single" myth. People are forced to be happy when they're single.

I didn't mind being single for a long time, to be honest. I made the most out of it. But what I mean is that you can never be complete if you're only half of the equation. *Yin* can't work without *yang*. They're both part of a whole while being completely different.

The same goes for relationships. We're not made to be single our whole lives. Just look at people who have bee single for the majority of their lives. They're mostly heavy drinkers. They mostly try to cover up something that they're missing, but you can't cover it up with alcohol.

229. THE IMPORTANCE OF AN OFF DAY

My off day used to be a Tuesday because we trained on Sundays. This was all sunshine and rainbows until I decided to pick up my training pace. I suddenly realized that Tuesday was a horrible day to take as an off day. I did have a lot of time to relax because I still had to go to my job.

I eventually changed camps and the first thing that I did was make sure that I took Sunday as my off day. In that way, I had a whole day to recharge my batteries mentally and physically. This approach really worked because it made me aware of the fact that there's a limit on the amount of energy that my body can generate. It just took some time to make myself aware of this. Don't make the same mistake I did.

230. WORK WITH WHAT YOU HAVE

I know an older woman who got divorced at a young age. She eventually met a really great guy, but there was one problem: he still had kids who went to high school, so they were forced to live in their own house. This all worked out until the woman suddenly wanted to break up because she wanted to be home more.

I know that it wasn't perfect to live apart together, but shouldn't you work with what you've got? There is no such thing as a perfect relationship. Every relationship will have certain things that'll make you rethink the whole thing.

But I mean, c'mon. Am I the only one who really thinks that this is stupid? Sounds like a great deal of fun to be home alone all the time. Gives you a lot of time to rethink your whole life and I'm pretty sure that thinking about that decision all the time can't be pleasant.

231. THE BEST ADVICE I'VE EVER GIVEN

You know what the best advice I ever gave? I didn't even give it to the guy. I never told the guy that he should quit his job, even though he was directly asking me to say so. He eventually quit his job and I was very happy for him, but I never gave him advice.

So many people like to give others advice. They constantly tell them what to do and what to say, but they forget one simple thing. They're dealing with another person who they're constantly instructing. It's really delusional and just prove how "empathic" people really are. They don't care about your problems. They just want to place themselves above you.

232. AN EASY WAY TO SOLVE (MOST OF) YOUR PROBLEMS

There's an easy hack to solve all your problems. Ever noticed that you're always so good at solving other people's problems but never yours? That's because they are emotionally attached to the problem and you're not. You can see the problem without a single emotion, which makes it easy to solve the problem.

Try to take the same approach. Try to look at your problem from a spectator's perspective. It makes most problems seem a lot smaller or almost irrelevant. I'm not claiming that this is applicable to all problems, but it'll seal the deal in 99% of the cases.

233. LISTEN TO COMPREHEND INSTEAD OF WITH THE INTENT TO REPLY

"**D**o you even listen?" I'll bet that most guys who've been in a relationship will recognize this sentence.

For the ones who have never heard it - congratulations, you're an emphatic listener. But most people are far from emphatic listeners. They listen with the intent to respond instead of the intent to listen. "How do you mean, Alex?" Good listening! Well, they don't ask questions to be able to talk about themselves. Those people's whole way of thinking is ego-driven. They only care about themselves. This results in the fact that these people aren't able to learn something new, but it doesn't stop there. It can kill your marriage, your friendships and so on.

You don't believe me, do you? Well, let me tell you a funny

Alex De Wilde

story...

234. YOU SHOULD BE CURIOUS INSTEAD OF JUDGMENTAL

I once wrote a blog post about the fact that you should approach life like a martial art. This basically meant that you should approach everything as if you are a white belt. You should be curious and open to learning new things.

So many people claim that things are impossible or that a certain person can't achieve something. Dream killers are extremely egocentric people. They assume that they know everything. They've got it all figured out. Well, that's their perception, of course. It's a sign that their thinking is ego-bound and a sign of stupidity as well. Let me share you a quote from one of the smartest people that's ever walked the Earth:

"The only thing I know is that I know nothing, and I am not quite sure that I know that." (Aristotle)

He was so smart, yet he still claimed that he knew nothing. Now that's a sign of intelligence.

235. MOST MODERN-DAY RELATIONSHIPS ARE DOOMED FROM THE START

Have you noticed that almost all the modern-day relationships are the same? There are some exceptions, but a lot of people are still in toxic relationships. The worst part is that they all assume that it's normal. It's a delusional way of thinking but it exists.

Those people tend to give advice to others and it mostly doesn't make any sense. The best "worst advice" that I've ever had was this:

"You only know if you're in a good relationship if you're fighting and arguing all the time."

I responded that I didn't want a good relationship if that was an indicator of the quality. I seriously even wonder how you can believe such a quote. That doesn't sound right, does it? But then it struck me. I suddenly realized where this misconception came from. You can never be in a good relationship if you've never seen a great example.

236. THE "THREE GENERATION" RULE THAT OCCURS OVER AND OVER AGAIN

The first generation is the generation that builds everything up. This was my grandparents' generation in which they survived the war. The second generation has more comfort and doesn't work that hard. The third generation doesn't work hard either because they never saw a great example from their parents. So what generation are we in now? The third one. So what happens after the third generation, you ask?

Things go to ruin and we will need start all over again. This is what happened to Rome. But we can change this dynamic simply by working hard. Society can't collapse if we don't get comfortable. There's just one problem. We're surrounded by a lot of comfort.

237. DO YOU HAVE A BUSY OR PRODUCTIVE LIFESTYLE? (PART I)

This may come as a shocker to you, but being busy doesn't equate to having a successful lifestyle. Most people assume that the busiest people are the most successful, but many of these people get nothing done. You can watch television all day, but that doesn't mean that you're going to get anything done.

Most people use the "I'm too busy" excuse way too often, in my opinion. You have to read between the lines when it comes to this one. Those people just don't consider it as a priority but use the "no time" excuse to cancel on you or flake out on other things. But this is the most common form of the no time excuse.

I've heard of way worse situations where people claimed that they couldn't get a single, simple thing done. The worst one I've seen was when someone was complaining that it was impossible to make his own bed. He didn't have time to do it.

How can't you make time to make up a bed? How long does it take? Thirty seconds?

238. DO YOU HAVE A BUSY OR A PRODUCTIVE LIFESTYLE? (PART II)

Another thing that I've noticed is that busy people are often chronic procrastinators. They just avoid the things that they should do and then suddenly have to do it all at once in a brief period of time. That's incredibly stressful, too. These people also often hate on me when I post a quote about wasting time because that's what most people do in the end. They waste a lot of time and then can't do what they actually wanted to do. So what's the main point here?

Do what you have to do today instead of tomorrow and you won't feel sorrow.

239. ARE YOU HARD TO GET OR JUST UNAVAILABLE?

A girl once asked me if I romantically availabe. I told her that I was, at least according to Facebook. She showed clear interest in me, yet I didn't respond to it. You know why? Because she didn't want to put in any effort.

But that's not the only point of this quote. The point is that a lot of women play the "hard to get" game and the results are mostly the opposite of what they want to achieve. I get it you don't want to be labeled as easy, but you have to draw a line somewhere. Some women really push it to the limit and guys just keep on chasing them. Crazy if you ask me. I've ditched girls who have acted like this rather quickly. I knew that they were up to no good.

So how do you know that you've found the right one? That's a great question, right? Let me explain the secret to finding "the one" in the next chapter...

240. READY TO MEET "THE ONE"?

The main thing you need to know when you want to meet "the one" is that two people who like each other will most likely spend more and more time together. That's the main idea: it comes naturally.

People always try to force things, but you can't force things. That'll never work out for the better; in fact, it'll mostly have the opposite effect. So that's the secret, which isn't actually a secret. It's common sense and that's the reason why most people can't figure it out. They lack common sense. They google "10 signs that a girl likes me" or "the best way to seduce a girl," but all that shit is completely irrelevant. I've done it and it has ruined dates because it's completely unnatural to look for these signs or use those pick-up artist tricks. It just comes naturally.

Someone once told me this and I assumed that he was lying. Turns out that he was completely right.

241. YOUR PRIORITIES NEED TO SHIFT FROM TIME TO TIME

Did you know that I stopped training for a week to get this book done? I was behind on schedule and needed to do it even though I really didn't like the idea of shifting my priorities around.

But this goes for everything in life. Sometimes you have to shift priorities and make something important and urgent. Finishing this book was really important to me because this was a way out of the rat race for me. People don't seem to get this concept. They always neglect what's important and do what's urgent.

Don't be like these people. Learn to be aware of the things that are important and prioritize these. A good example of this is a couple who starts to fight and keeps on fighting beyond bedtime. Going to bed might be urgent, but solving the matter is important.. Get it? Good!

242. THE MAIN THING IS TO KEEP THE MAIN THING THE MAIN THING

My main thing is and will remain MMA. That'll be like that until I hit my late 30s. MMA has remained the main thing during my last whole week. I study the sport extensively at my job to get a better understand of certain things. Because deep down, I was pretty pissed that I couldn't train.

During this whole period, I reminded myself that the week after, I needed to get this book finished and that I had to pick up training again. You can only be really good at one thing. All the other things are just distracting from the main goal. So the main thing is to keep the main thing the main thing.

243. MY DAD CALLED ME "OBSESSED." I THANKED HIM AND HE DIDN'T GET IT.

My dad once called me "obsessed" because I was watching some MMA breakdown right after I had finished my second training session of the day. He did it to insult me and likely to get on my nerves. His intentions were confusing, to be honest. But he didn't get why I thanked him or why the whole insult didn't affect me.

Realize this: people will try to insult you every single day, but most of their insults can be turned into a compliment. I'm really obsessed, but this just proves that I'm not all about the talk - I actually walk the walk. People notice this and take notes. Some like it and others don't, but that's just a matter of where their mindset lies.

244. MIRROR, MIRROR ON THE WALL, WHO PROJECTS INSECURITIES ON THEM ALL?

People who hate on others mostly project their own insecurities onto them.

You might not believe me, but this is an actually true story. There was a woman who once claimed that I had no vision whatsoever in life and that I was a failure as well. I didn't udnerstand why she said this until I took a closer look at the women's life. She had no vision in life and she also hadn't achieved anything she wanted. So she was projecting all those things onto me.

That's pretty absurd, if you ask me. But it's also a tool that you know this because now you can take the upper hand. I replied calmly, "that's cute, but you're projecting your own insecurities onto me." She immediately started to defend herself, trying to prove me wrong. She was like the insecure weakling who got called out. Bullseye.

245. ALWAYS GIVE SOMETHING BACK IN LIFE.

I realized something when I finally beat my depression. I realized that I was blessed to still be alive. I realized that I had a gift and a story, and now it was time to share this story. That's the thing that most people lack these days. They take everything for granted and just worship themselves in the mirror.

It's extremely important to avoid being so egocentric and actually help people. From time to time, people who are my age have contacted me to tell me that they have been through similar stuff and that they were happy that I shared my story. It always feel nice when people tell me stuff like this. It makes me want to do it even more. Everybody has a story and everybody can help out other people. The question is if you're actually going to do it.

246. CAN YOUR PHONE RUIN YOUR WHOLE LIFE?

The smartphone has become a big part of our lives. I admit that it's so convenient to have a camera, music player, GPS, and so much more all in one, but that doesn't mean that the damn thing should be glued to your hands.

Focus more on your friends than on your phone and you'll notice that you'll have a lot more fun in conversations. I mean, it's pretty boring to talk about what others post on Facebook or Instagram, isn't it? I noticed that this is a very popular topic among friends these days. Stop focusing on others and start focusing on what really matters.

To add onto that, you should never text and drive. You're not so important that you have the right to text while behind the wheel. Give others' lives the same value as you give your own.

247. HOW TO HANDLE REJECTION LIKE A GENTLEMAN

I had a match after three swipes once on Tinder. She was my type for sure. We started talking and she soon asked about my blog. It was a fun conversation, so I asked her to meet up. I didn't have any expectations. I just planned to go there, have fun and see what happens. We kept on talking for a few days, but two days before the big day, she told me that she wasn't ready to date.

I wasn't mad at her. I even thanked her for being so honest. She was surprised by my reaction, which is normal, I guess. Rejecting someone isn't fun and a bit stressful as well. Those people are afraid of the reaction of the other person. You don't want to offend someone for being honest.

So why was I able to process it so easily? Well, that's because life goes on no matter what. Tomorrow, there's just another day. I just didn't see a reason to get mad. I even hope that she meets the right person.

248. HOW TO GET THE MOST OUT OF YOUR WEEK OFF.

The answer is pretty simple: rest while remaining active at the same time! Just get up early, walk or walk your dog, read some books, spend time with friends, and so on. An off week means that you're actually taking time off and not that you're going to put in any more work.

In addition, you should be aware of the fact that you can easily overeat during this period. The main goal of this week is to recharge the batteries. So rest, read and recover. Sound pretty easy, right? You can do it! No work or other projects allowed!

249. DEVELOP AN IRON WILL BECAUSE IT'S AN EASY SKILL

P eople often claim that they'll be trying to do something. That's cute, but you have to actually do that something. Don't try - just do it. Trying leads to crying. It's that simple.

People who "try" stuff aren't 100% confident that they'll actually be able to pull it off. So they fail because they weren't committed right from the start.

Also, they will ease their minds afterwards by telling themselves, "well, at least you tried." I really hate that sentence. We should encourage these people to do it again, and again, and again until they succeed. There are more things that will make you increase your willpower, but this one is a major tip to get started.

250. THE ONLY THING THAT'S IMPOSSIBLE IN LIFE

There's only one thing that's impossible in life. Well, actually two, since you'll never own a dinosaur as a pet. You're probably disappointed about this; I had the same feeling when I heard the news that I couldn't own a dinosaur.

OK, enough joking. What's really impossible? Can you name something that seems impossible in your opinion? The answer is actually simple: the only thing that's impossible is to beat a person who doesn't want to give up. It's really impossible to do. They have such strong self- belief that you're drawn to them. They even make you relive all your childhood dreams. Cool, isn't it?

Now get ready for some #instamotivation.

251. NOTHING IS IMPOSSIBLE

Have you ever read *Mediations*, the famous book written by Marcus Aurelius? This book was written before the time of Christ and the author already knew the value of hardwork and self-belief. He thought that nothing was impossible if you just put in the time and work.

Many people claim that talent does exist, but they're denying the hard work that others put in. Well, it's that but also the fact that they're too afraid to do something themselves. They're just easing their minds and accepting the fact that they are lazy.

Nobody just wants to accept that they're lazy. Stop making excuses and start accomplishing shit. I really hate when people make excuses all the time. Get your life in check and stop whining. Not a single problem was solved by complaining about it and not a single thing was accomplished by doing nothing.

Do you get it? You do? So why are still reading this and not pursuing what you really want? Get up and do something, because nothing impossible.

252. YOU'RE A PIECE OF SHIT IF YOU LAUGH WHEN PEOPLE GET HIT

So I got kicked in the nose in training. I've never seen so much blood coming out of a nose before. The blood was running for about 15 minutes. It wasn't pretty to see. We all assumed that it was broken, but luckily it wasn't. So I took a selfie and put it on my Snapchat story.

I didn't want pity or anything like that. I didn't need a reaction at all. But some people mocked me or laughed at me. I was like, "What kind of sick person are you that you laugh with someone who got hit in the face?" That's pretty sick, right? I suggest that you really work on yourself if you don't understand this.

The sad part is that those people don't even realize how twisted that really is. They focus on other people because they don't want to face their own demons. That's just a sad reality.

253. THE BASICS ARE CRUCIAL, WHICH IS WHAT MOST PEOPLE FORGET

L et's talk about "the basics" in life for a minute. Most people hate the basics. Can you guess why? Because they all assume the basics are boring. Well, the thing is that the basics are easy and not fancy at all. But they work and you need to understand that you won't achieve anything in life for you if you neglect them.

I recently watched a training video by John Wayne Parr. He's a Muay Thai legend. In the video, he was drilling the jab and double jab over and over again. It's basically the first punch you learn. I got why he did it like this, but so many people were bitching about it. They all assumed that he trained way more fancy shit and that he didn't want to give away his training secrets. Well, he gave them away but most people were too ignorant to realize it.

Oh, "normal" people. You continue to be so entertaining.

254. STOP LOOKING FOR SHORTCUTS

People are looking for shortcuts all the time. What's more, I noticed that the smartest people tend to do it the most. I mean people with a ton of degrees. They want to be rich and famous, but they just can't figure out how to do it.

So what do they do? They search for shortcuts their whole damn lives. And at some point, they start feeling cheated by life. They constantly blame everything and everyone. That's all they do. Those people don't take ownership of their own life and mistakes. They act like pussies and they don't even realize it.

"So Alex, are there really no shortcuts?" Well, you could sell drugs, but you'd probably end up in jail or dead. Playing the lottery will eventually lose everything you own, so that's not an option either. So what do you have to do then? Well...

255. THERE ARE NO SHORTCUTS FOR HARD WORK

You can't substitute hard work. You have to work for everything if you're serious about it!

"But Alex, I don't like hard work." Well, enjoy going to your dead-end job, my friend. Enjoy being out of shape for the rest of your life. You can come up with tons of excuses as to why you haven't achieved something, but you just fucked up - that's it. You played tons of video games instead of working out. All that unhealthy food didn't help either.

Let me set something straight. You, and nobody else is responsible for what you achieve in life. So you either look for shortcuts all the time or you just work and that's it.

Go after what you want. It's not impossible! You've just got to pull the trigger.

256. "ONE MORE TIME" DOESN'T SOLVE YOUR WORRIES ON A DIME

There are a lot of people who live lives that could be part of a reality show. These are also the people who like to watch reality shows, funnily enough. It's pretty logical since they just want to laugh at other people's pain to forget their own.

These people don't get that they inflict all this drama onto themselves. I mean, they make their choices and nobody else does it for them, right? Those people haven't got a single clue what they want and like in life. They usually don't even have their own identity. They're a stranger to themselves. So they always give people "one more time" when those people hurt them. Can you guess what this means? They still have an unlimited amount of strikes before they're out.

These people get hurt all the time because nobody takes them seriously. It's like a full-time profession to them. The sad part is that they don't take action. They always ask, "why always me?: Zero problems are solved by asking that question.

257. TWO STRIKES AND YOU'RE OUT

This hack makes life a lot easier. People often give others unlimited chances, but that doesn't include me and it shouldn't include you either. You can try to pull off something with me twice, but you're out after that.

There have been a lot of people in my life who have assumed that this wouldn't happen to me. So they tried to pull off some kind of terrible behavior on me. Those people didn't take the warning seriously the first time, so they were given the boot after the second time. No hard feelings, but those people will never be a part of my life again.

Two strikes is what it takes. You see, I have clear boundaries and people better not try to pass them. I clearly tell people when they've crossed the line. I'm not afraid to get out of my comfort zone and confront people about their behavior. Some people are just full of shit or too dumb to care about you. That's why I used this principle.

258. WHY ONLY TWO STRIKES ALEX?

Because most people never really change. They get a warning the first time and are surprised that I really made my boundaries clear. Most of the time, they just improve their way of lying instead of their mindset. This is the sad reality for most of the people.

I don't know that many people who've changed for the better, to be honest. Most of them just got dumber and dumber. That's why I make sure that I never give a third chance. They'd mostly fuck it up anyways, so it would be a waste of time.

To this day, on I've never met a person that did something bad only once. This is a sad reality, but it's really good that you know things like this. They make life easier. I suggest you pick up *Laws Of Human Nature* by Robert Greene to dive deeper on this topic.

259. THE BIG "WHAT IF" SHOW

"But Alex, what if they really change after the second strike?"

That's a possibility, of course. There are two options here. You either meet again or just never know. But I seriously wonder why you would even think about this choice. Just be present in the moment and see what happens.

I wish all the people that I have removed from my life the best, but I'm not focused on what they're doing. It's safe to say that I actually don't care, to be honest. I have stuff of my own to take care of. I'm focusing on what matters in life. Focusing on others is not important to me. That's just a big waste of time. None of this would have happened if they didn't step my boundaries in the first place.

260. DEVELOP AN "ALPHA MENTALITY"

I get up every single day with the thought that I'm a zero. I start back at square one and I have one simple mission. It's pretty easy to be honest: I just want to beat myself. I want to do better than I did the day before. I want to become a better person by the end of the day. The alpha mentality is all about evolving to the best version of yourself.

Now I know that people will have some questions about this. They ask stuff like, "is it hard?" Nothing is hard if you like doing it. Hard work is the best thing there is but only if you're working towards something meaningful. That's it. I use this mindset in training, blogging and elsewhere in my life. Get better or get bitter, I say, and I don't want to get bitter, so I just become better every single day.

Or "the more you sweat, the luckier you are," as I like to say. Sounds pretty badass, doesn't it? I know you want to retweet it. Go ahead! Just tweet it!

261. LIFE IS ALL ABOUT CREATING MOMENTUM

You need to create momentum in order to get something out of life. But you'll have to create it in everything that you do. You can't expect tons of results from short-term intensity. You have to have long-term consistency.

How do you create long-term consistency, you ask? By creating momentum. It's even a law in physics: "an object at rest stays at rest, and an object in motion stays in motion with the same speed and in the same direction unless acted upon by an unbalanced force." This is called Newton's First Law. There's a lot of truth in this law and most people don't seem to get it at all. They're an object for sure, but they're not moving at all.

You can't expect a couch potato to do great things. They eat chips in front of the television and that's all. Those are the people who hate others because they're jealous of their achievements. You haven't created momentum, so you can't bitch about it.

262. ARE SACRIFICES NECESSARY TO ACHIEVE THINGS?

I really like it when people tell me that they want to be successful but don't want to make all the sacrifices. I'm like, "what do you mean with sacrifices?" Most people claim that they'll miss their favorite television shows, for example. Interesting, isn't it? They want to be successful, but they don't want to give up comfort. So here's what's going to happen: nothing.

There's no such thing as a sacrifice if you do what you really love. You're doing the wrong thing if you have to choose between what you proclaim that you want and something like going out or bingeing television shows and so on. That's it if you ask me. It doesn't feel like a sacrifice to me when I had to go to bed early on a Saturday night because I had grappling on Sunday morning. But I feel like I'm sacrificing sleep when I go out. It's all about priorities. So, sacrifices? I don't think so!

263. NO TIME? THAT EXCUSE IS PURE BULLSHIT.

So many people use the "no time" excuse to cancel plans. Too many people accept this dumb excuse, but I don't and I know other people who hate it as well.

The excuse is bullshit. People who use this excuse all the time are either pussies or they've lost their grip on life. I believe that it's safe to say that this is the cheapest excuse in our modern-day society. It really can't get any worse than this.

I remember a guy who once asked me how to get in shape. So I wanted to help him. Turns out that he had no time to cook or work out, but he did find plenty of time to be lazy. Funny, isn't it?

People who use this excuse are miserable, lazy or uninspired. That's why I had to debunk this once and for all. "No time" means "no priority." Change that!

264. CAN YOU GUESS THE DEFINITION OF "HELL"?

What is "hell"? You probably assume that hell must be something like being together with your ex again, but it's not.

The real definition of hell is this: on your last day on Earth, the person you became will meet the person you should have become.

Get it? Let it sink in for a moment. Now read it again. That's what I call a meaningful quote.

Can you even imagine that you meet yourself but as a better version. You'll suddenly realize that you fucked up your whole life. That can't be a joyful feeling and you can't escape death, so what can you do to avoid something like this? You just live your life. It's really that easy.

265. LEARN FROM OTHER PEOPLE'S REGRETS

Most people reflect on their lives when they realize that they're going to die. There are five common regrets that show up over and over again:

"I wish I'd had the courage to live a life true to myself, not the life others expected of me."

"I wish I hadn't worked so hard."

"I wish I'd had the courage to express my feelings."

"I wish I had stayed in touch with my friends."

"I wish that I had let myself be happier."

Memorize these regrets and make sure that you never face them. You might still have time to make a change while others are facing the pain of regret right now. We're all going to die, so why not die joyful?

266. TOMORROW THERE'S JUST ANOTHER NEW DAY (PART I)

I can't recall how many times that I've told this story so far, but it's the perfect way to prove a point.

I was going to a movie night with some friends. We ended up with three of us - two guys including me and a girl. We started watching a trilogy pretty late. The girl had seen the movies, so she was talking all the time about a past relationship. Well, she wasn't exactly talking about it. In fact, she kept complaining about it. You can't imagine how many problems a single person can have.

Anyway, I fell asleep somewhere during the second movie, but the last thing that I remember was the girl who complained about her ex. Here's where it gets crazy: she slept on the other side of the room, but I think that we woke up around the same time. Can you guess what she did? No "good morning" or anything. She just picked up where she left off, complaining about her ex. I was like, "you've just slept eight hours and you still have problems to complain about first thing in the morning?!"

267. TOMORROW THERE'S JUST ANOTHER NEW DAY (PART II)

Do you realize what I was trying to tell you with this story? Here's what you should realize: it doesn't matter what happened yesterday or even the day before. What matters the most is that you're present in the moment and make the most out of it.

Most people like to complain frequently, but that's just a waste of time. All your excuses will make sure that you never grow. Everybody will start to avoid you after a while. It's also weak behavior since you're not taking ownership of your life.

Let's take a look at the fact that the girl was complaining again. Did her ex do something bad to her very recently? No, he didn't, since she had been sleeping for the last eight hours.

Some people get stuck in the past and complain about irrelevant stuff. You need to master the art of "not giving a fuck." Take care of the things that you can control and forget about the stuff that you can't control.

268. ARE YOU CRAVING THE WEEKEND? THAT'S NO BUENO.

So most people set their alarm clock an hour early. They snooze for an hour and then get up. They eat some unhealthy food (though some eat healthy) and rush to work. Don't forget to spill the coffee! Then they get stuck in traffic and complain about the fact that they're in traffic. They go to a job that they hate but keep on doing it to make the money that they spend way too easily during the weekends.

Gossip and complaining about life are the topics at lunch, of course. The job ends at 5:00 and they go to the gym after, doing the same routine that they always do. It doesn't work at all, but they keep on doing it. Then they waste some time in front of television or on social media and finally go to sleep. Others go home and watch television until they have to go to sleep. They repeat the sequence the next day, offcourse, since there's nothing better than staying in your comfort zone.

269. THE WEEKEND IS EXTREMELY OVERRATED

There, I said it, and there's a good reason why I said it. People sleep until noon, so they waste half a day just by sleeping. They claim that they're tired, but they're not tired! They are uninspired! You have no clear goal in life, so you've got not a single reason to get up first thing in the morning.

So most people work a bit around the house and then they either watch television until they fall asleep or go out. They go out because they need to drink away their problems. They're actually drinking away their capability to think, but who am I to judge. Sundays are mostly the same besides the fact that most people spend an hour complaining that they have to return to work on Monday.

Somebody really has to explain to me why it's so much better to sleep all day long and just do nothing afterward. Are you even surprised that you're tired all the time? I'm not.

270. MOST PEOPLE LOVE AND HATE THE WEEKEND AT THE SAME TIME

I noticed that most people have a love/hate relationship with the weekend. They love it because they can sleep as long as they want, which sound pretty depressing if you ask me. I mean, you're going to die one day and you spend your time in a job you hate, in front of the television or sleeping in bed. Are you really happy? Don't pretend because you won't gain anything from it.

Most people love the weekend because they don't have to go to their job, but they hate it because they've got so much spare time. The struggle must be real since some of them would like to work on the weekends because they have nothing to do. It's actually pretty sad.

I hope that you realize that you'll live like this until you reach the age of retirement. This conclusion is a pretty painful reality check. Do you feel cheated by life already?

271. CHEERS TO THE FUCKING WEEKEND

So how do you get most out of your weekends? Well, you could start by getting up at the same time as you do on every other day of the week. You'll feel more energized because you didn't sleep in too late. Now you'll have a pretty long day.

Scared? Why? Because you've got so much time? That's actually a great thing. I usually write four blog posts, train twice and read a lot while I have time to relax on those two days. I advise you to read during the weekends, too. You'll become smarter in no time if you read every day.

Be active. Buy yourself a boxing bag and have some fun with that. You'll feel a lot better, trust me. Everybody likes hitting the bag. Find something you really like and spend your time doing that. Learn a new instrument, a new hobby, write a book... The options are endless. Just do something you like so don't you don't have to sleep all day. Easy-peasy, right?

272. UNHAPPINESS CAN MAKE YOU DO GREAT THINGS

Most people are extremely insecure about their appearance or potential. This combination can be a killer and is something that needs to be addressed as soon as possible. It's all in your head; that's something that most people don't even realize.

The person who says "I can" and the person who says "I can't" are both usually right. Sounds like a dumb motivational line, but it's correct. You poison your mind by telling yourself you can't and this results in the fact that you fail. The worst part is that you get a completely inaccurate image of yourself because you're lowering your self-esteem every damn time you do this.

It would be pretty dumb to ignore this fact and pretty damn foolish to keep on doing it. It's always better to make a change, but are you prepared to do it? Your mind is the most powerful supplement on the Earth.

273. WHAT DOESN'T KILL YOU MAKES YOU STRONGER

L ife is all about perception. You can label a situation as either good or bad. So learn to master the art of turning the odds into your favor. What doesn't kill you really makes you stronger.

Most people die mentally after a setback. Not literally, of course, but most people never recover from this setback. This is something that shouldn't occur in this day and age anymore. Those people don't realize that the cure for the pain is always within the pain.

This may be a lot to understand but realize that it's a long process. Change never happens overnight. Unhappiness should be your stepping stone and not something that holds you down.

274. STUCK IN A RUT? FOLLOW YOUR GUT!

W hat's a gut feeling, you ask? Your gut feeling is the initial reaction to a certain situation. It'll tell you if you're on the right path or not. But most people lose this feeling over time. They don't trust their own intuition anymore. Instead they rely on other people's opinions or even statistics that are shared by the media. I can draw two conclusions from the previous sentence.

(1)   The person clearly doesn't believe in himself anymore.
(2)   He needs statistics to prove that he can't do something.

I don't care about statistics and other people's opinions. They all act like experts, but their advice mostly sucks. The advice that has been given before it's asked is often terrible. Smart people don't give advice until they're asked to give it. Can you guess what I do? I just believe in myself and there's not a single statistic that'll be able to change it. So where do most people go wrong?

275. WHERE MOST PEOPLE FAIL IS BEFORE THEY EVEN START

Go stand in front of a mirror and take a good look. Have you done it? Well, you've just seen your biggest competitor. You only have to compete with yourself and no one else.

You should follow your gut feeling instead of overthinking everything. If you don't, you'll have tons of choices and then you'll have tons of different outcomes. You'll never be able to choose.

Just make a decision and make sure that it turns out great. The right decision isn't always right from the start. You're only going to regret a certain decision if you made a lot of bad choices after the initial one. Those will make sure that you end up in a worse situation than before. That's why you're stuck in a rut. The sad part is that you'll probably be stuck in your own head as well.

276. FOLLOW YOUR GUT OR KEEP YOUR MOUTH SHUT

It'll be hard to turn your life around. I'm not going to lie about it and it'll only get harder the longer you wait. You'll just come up with more scenarios and outcomes, but there's a certain action that's a lot more dangerous. You could calm yourself and convince yourself that things will get better over time.

I hate to break it to you, but they won't. Nothing will get better if you don't take action. It's all up to you to take the first step to a new and better life. People will judge you, but those are the ones who were afraid to do it themselves. Don't mind them. Do what you need to do.

"So what do I have to do, Alex?" You have to make yourself happy because no one else will do it for you!

277. SAVE YOUR DRAMA FOR YOUR MAMA

This was actually a quote that I used to point out that someone was whining. Yeah, I wasn't shy to throw around some fancy one-liners when I was attending my last year in college. I still do it to this day.

Now, to all the little boys who cause a lot of drama: step up, shut up and man the fuck up. I don't care if you're doing it in real life or on social media. It needs to stop right now. Don't be part of our pussy generation. You're causing a lot of unnecessary problems for other people.

People have important stuff to do and your little ego isn't important at all. Welcome to the way of the alpha. Thank you and don't come again. Drama isn't for sale.

278. SO TELL ME AGAIN: WHY ARE YOU WAITING ON THE PERFECT MONDAY?

I always wonder why people ditch the whole plan when it doesn't work out. I get that you want to change your life, but do you really want it? Be honest with yourself; I might shock you out of your illusion in a minute.

You see, most people believe that they want something, but in reality they don't want it. They just want comfort. That's where it all goes wrong, since you can't have both. You can't stay in your comfort zone and make a drastic change in your life. Some people just don't seem to realize this. But I hope that you get it now? Good, because I'm not done yet.

279. DO YOU REALLY WANT IT? I DON'T THINK SO.

Most people don't want the change badly enough. I mean, why would you wait until Monday to make a new start? That's just bullshit. People who really want something start right away. You're already failing before you've even started.

You can make tons of great plans, but they won't always work out. Let's assume that you start your perfect plan by getting up early. What if you can't get up and fall asleep again? Will you wait another week before you try it again? Will you give in to all the bad habits that kill your happiness in the first place? You can fuck up a lot in seven days.

People who fail to start often have a list of excuses a well. These excuses make sure they never grow. It's like they write a list of excuses and a perfect plan at the same time. That would be a big waste of time!

280. BALANCE IS THE KEY TO A HAPPY LIFE

You want to have a happy life, don't you? Well, you'll need to be able to find balance. But I can guarantee you that it's harder than it seems. It's easy to write about it, but finding the balance itself is harder at times.

You see, life is just a series of highs (happy times) and lows (less pleasant times). Some people get caught up in the lows and those people get stuck in a rut. Those are the people who feel cheated by life. Life, however, didn't cheat them; those people cheated on their selves. They couldn't find balance, so they fell down and never got up.

It's not their fault. They just don't teach you this stuff in school. Luckily, I'm here to help you. The following three chapters will help you big time.

281. LIFE & THE QUEST TO FIND BALANCE

L ife is like playing the piano. The white keys represent happiness and the black keys sadness or hard times. But as you go through life's journey, remember that the black keys also make music.

The key (get it?) to finding balance in life is not getting caught up in the highs and the lows. Both are dangerous to be stuck in. A high or multiple highs are mostly followed by one or multiple lows. So you'll be even hit harder if you're assuming that you won't face adversity. But I get it. It's easy to assume that you can handle the world when life's going great. It's at that point that you'll face the bad times.

The people who are stuck in a negative mindset will do stupid things due to their unhappiness. Those people need to be able to turn things around and that's only possible when you take action.

282. IT'S GOOD, IT'S BAD, IT'S A LITTLE BIT OF BOTH

Life isn't good or bad. Things that happen to you aren't good or bad. Life is whatever you make from it. It's all about perception.

I had some highs a while ago and I felt great. A bit too great, to be honest. I really got caught up in it. The lows followed quickly after and I was smart enough to realize that I was getting caught up in them. I addressed the lows and made sure that I could find balance again.

You can only get out of the bad times if you learn a lesson from those times. That's when you learn to appreciate them. I haven't found a low to this day onward which didn't teach me a lesson. This actually means that you'll be learning new things about yourself non-stop.

283. BALANCE & LEARNING

People don't seem to get how I learn lessons from the bad times. Well, it's pretty easy. I just reflect on stuff. I look back at a time when I faced a low and think about what I did/said and what happened. Sometimes you won't solve it directly. I've solved issues months after they happened, but I always solved them.

You've got a brain, so why don't you start using it? Oh, I know why. You're braindead because you feed your brain nothing useful. You won't become any smarter by watching television or spending all your time on social media.

Remember that I told you that life is like playing the piano? You need to bad times in order to grow and enjoy the good times. So why don't you sit down and start playing a tune? Just make sure that you strike the black keys, too.

284. THE REASON WHY YOU'RE FACING REGRET

It's pretty simple, to be honest. You take an action and it doesn't work out as you imagined it. So you end up in a worse situation than before you took that certain action. Now you're craving the time where things were better." You don't realize that those times only look better in retrospect. That's it.

That's the reason why people return to past relationships, shitty jobs or even college. There are a lot of college dropouts who return just because they can't get their lives together. The sad part is that most people judge those people while they would probably do the same thing in their situation.

285. TAKE THE BET AND BEAT REGRET

L et me share with you some life wisdom: you won't always take the right decision, but that doesn't mean that you can't make the decision right. Get it?

It's all about your actions after you make a certain decision. For example, work on yourself after a breakup. Make sure that you get a better job after you quit your previous one. Go all-in if you do something. Don't try something but do something! I'm a college dropout and there wasn't a single point in time where I even considered going back. I hated it and I'm a lot happier now, but that wouldn't have happened if I didn't work on myself. It was and still is one of the best decisions that I ever took.

I really didn't expect that it would turn out like this, but I was willing to step out of my comfort zone. It's all about hard work. I took an action but I also made sure that it would turn out great. I wanted to prove to myself that I could turn a "bad situation" into a good one.

286. THE MAGIC
OF WORDS

Did you know that there's magic in your words? Most people don't realize this, but you can speak things into existence. You can make something happen if you say it many times.

The perfect example is the person who constantly claims that they'll be sick tomorrow. Guess what happens the day after? They get sick and then they'll be like, "See? I told you so."

So what do we have to do if we realize that our words can make us sick? We have to watch our words. Saying things like "I'm depressed" too often will make you depressed. The same goes for when you're about to give up in training. Don't say "I have to give up." Say something like "I'm going to get through this, the pain is just temporary."

Your attitude determines your altitude, so watch your words. You'll remain a loser if you keep claiming that you're a loser.

287. THE MAGIC OF WORDS? FEED THE HOLLOW ONES TO THE BIRDS.

I had a good friend once who claimed that she wanted to meet up with me before I traveled to Stockholm. So I told her that I could schedule her in a week before I left. She just gave tons of excuses about things that she had to do. We never did end up meeting.

It wasn't until six months later that we were going to meet again. Guess what happened? She pulled the same shit on me!

People like to delude themselves and others with how busy they are because it makes them look successful. It's bullshit. Don't say things that aren't true because now she lives up to those things. She isn't as productive as she used to be. She's gotten busy instead of productive.

Don't say things that can ruin your life and don't say things that will ruin your progress! It's so dangerous. Who wants to get create momentum and then lose it again? Really stupid if you ask me.

288. CALL PEOPLE OUT ON THEIR BULLSHIT

Remember the girl from the previous chapter? I let it slide the first time, but I called her out the second time. She doesn't have a job, so she has 16 hours per day to be productive. I just told her that she has eight hours more than me in a day and that she should use them better.

I really don't care about people's excuses because they're just undermining their own potential. There are professional fighters who work two jobs, train four hours a day, and they still find the time to be with friends, family and loved ones. I have a job and train 17 hours a week, plus I run a podcast, a blog and a YouTube channel. What the fuck is your excuse?

So tell people when they're making excuses. They're blocking their own potential. This is sad but true. They might ignore you for the rest of their lives, but at least you did your job. You lift people up or you leave them behind if they don't want to be lifted up.

289. THE MAGIC OF THOUGHTS

We all face random thoughts throughout the day and some even don't make sense. I mean, have you ever thought something and wondered where it was coming from? Nobody is safe from these things, yet some people act on these thoughts while others don't.

There's a secret to this. They call this the "observant mind" in Buddhism. You observe thoughts but don't give any attention to them. It's like watching traffic. The thoughts pass by and you just let them pass.

Now, can you guess what happens when you stop a thought? You give it a lot of power, probably even more than it should get and then all the others don't have time to come through. The thought that you've picked might be one that's just an illusion that your mind created. We all face these thoughts so let them pass. They don't do you any good.

"Be careful what you think, because your thoughts run your life." (Proverbs, 4:23)

290. TAKE THE BET, PICK A GOAL TO SET

Did you know that I write down what I want to achieve at the end of every year? I write down a lot of things and some things aren't even realistic, but I still try to achieve them.

I wrote down two years in a row that I wanted to fight and that I wanted to meet the woman of my dreams. It took me just two years to achieve these goals. The thing that you have to realize is that you can't achieve everything at once. What I mean is that you might face stumbling blocks before you actually achieve them. So pick things that you really want and write them down again next year if you didn't achieve them. It doesn't matter when you achieve them. What matters is that you achieve them.

291. BEING CHEAP IS A VERY EXPENSIVE LIFESTYLE

People are always worried about money. They can't live without it and that's where the problem lies. People mostly buy stuff that they don't need because it makes them happy, or at least that's what they assume. But it doesn't make them happy; it makes sure that they go broke at a rapid pace. But then they suddenly realize that they have to buy food as well. So they buy the cheapest food and claim that they'll be fine.

This works for a while and maybe even for many years, but the small damage that you did will worsen over time. You'll be sick a lot and might even become extremely sick. So in the end, cheap people have to live an expensive lifestyle. They save on food, but they quickly spend all their money at the hospital. This is sad, so remember this one simple thing: "health is wealth." You don't need that $500 pair of headphones, but you do need to eat healthy. So do the right thing.

292. YOU'LL START TO FADE IF YOU'RE NOT MENTALLY CHALLENGED

Remember that I worked in a meat factory? I did this for four months and can guess what happened? All my blog posts made during that period weren't that great, to be honest. The job was boring and repetitive, and I frequently had to deal with brain fog during the day. I was starting to get dumber and dumber with every single minute that I spent there because I wasn't challenging myself.

The same goes for people who have a desk job. It's a soul-killing job that puts you to sleep. You're exhausted when you go home, but think about it. Have you ever been dead tired when you practiced sports or did something productive? You weren't so tired, right? Your body is giving you signals that you're doing the wrong thing and you're not listening to it. You just keep on doing it because you're too lazy to take action or you're so far gone that you don't believe in yourself anymore.

293. PEOPLE KEEP TELLING ME THAT I'VE CHANGED. I TELL THEM THAT THEY'RE STILL THE SAME.

Someone once tried to insult me by telling me that I had changed. I didn't feel hurt because it wasn't an insult to me. This was a compliment from someone who hadn't changed at all.

People mostly assume that change is a bad thing, but it isn't. They just want you to stay the same because they don't want to change or they want to use you like in the old days. This person in particular was someone that used to walk over me all the time, but times have changed and it doesn't happen anymore.

The "you've changed basically means that they can't cope with the fact that they can't use you anymore. So I tell people that they're still the same when they tell me that I've changed. There's one question that remains: who insults who?

294. YOU'LL FACE HATERS WHEN YOU TAKE ACTION. YOU'LL FACE REGRET WHEN YOU DON'T TAKE ACTION. PICK YOUR POISON.

Some people want to take action, but they're afraid of the haters. They face inevitable regret because they didn't take action. It's a never-ending cycle until you pick your poison. You're either going to face regret or you're going to face haters.

Both of them might suck, but facing haters is a lot easier than facing regret. Well, at least in my opinion. You know why? Because you can still get something out of life when you face haters. You're may even be doing the right thing if people hate on you. Regret, on the other hand, is a little bit tougher because that means that it's probably too late to change the outcome. So take action because regret tends to kill people slowly.

295. MOST PEOPLE WILL DO ANYTHING TO GET IN SHAPE

They'll do everything to get in shape, alright, but they'll skip on the eating clean and working hard parts. I've met so many people over the years who have wanted to be in shape and most of them failed because they always wanted to take the easy route.

Some people eat french fries all day while taking fat burners and barely working out. They take meal replacement shakes instead of actually eating healthy and then combined that with those seven-minute workouts. See what I mean? People want to spend millions on personal trainers while they don't want to work out. They spend tons of money on dieticians while they already know what they have to do.

It's like they're spending all this money just to wait and pull the "bad genetics" card to convince people that they just can't do it. Well, you can do it, but you have to work hard and eat clean. That's it.

296. AGE IS EITHER A NUMBER OR AN EXCUSE

People tend to claim that they're too young or to old, but the reality is that your age doesn't matter. Age is just a number and people need to start realizing this.

I once met a guy who wanted to start grappling, but he claimed that he was too old. He was 23 at the time, which is extremely young. Life hasn't even started yet and you're already coming up with excuses. That's a bit weird, isn't it?

Be smart about how you deal with those things. The best time to start is right now. Your age is just irrelevant. Somehow I wonder how people can convince themselves that they're too old when they're just in their twenties. I mean, what are you going to do when you hit your sixties? Some people even claim that you're not old at that age. I've got a wrestling trainer who's 64 and he still beats all the young guys. What's your excuse?

297. PEOPLE ALWAYS FIND AN EXCUSE TO JUDGE OTHERS BUT NEVER TO BETTER THEMSELVES

This is actually something that I noticed over time. People like to judge others because it's the easy way out and people like to take the path of least resistance.

It's obvious that it's a lot easier to judge others than to work on ourselves. This is actually weird as well because those people should find tons of reasons to better themselves, but somehow they just can't. Why don't they find them? Because they're not honest with themselves. They're so delusional that they assume that they're perfect while being from it. It's delusional to even assume that you can reach perfection.

So why don't you take a close look in the mirror next time you try to judge others. Why don't you try to see in what areas that you can improve. The path of least resistance is mostly a cursed path. Do I need to say more?

298. GO YOUR OWN WAY BECAUSE THE RIGHT PEOPLE WILL STAY AND THE WRONG PEOPLE WILL GO AWAY

At one point in time, you'll find out who really wants the best for you. A lot of people claim that they want you to do better in life until you actually start doing better. That's when so-called friends will turn on you, family members will turn their back on you ,and suddenly people of which you weren't even aware will start supporting you. It's a weird occurrence because you really can't predict who'll stay. Well, at least not at first.

The ones who stay are the ones who actually work on themselves. The others don't get better and don't want you to get better either. Learn from this and be aware of who'll support you and who won't. You should even be careful with the ones who won't support you because they might try to sabotage you. This might sound surreal until it actually happens to you.

299. ACTION IS THE HIGHWAY TO CONFIDENCE. WAITING IS THE HIGHWAY TO SELF-DOUBT.

People don't get that you can only become more confident by taking action. I once had a guy claim on Instagram that he wanted to be like me. He wanted to be where I was at after two years of constantly taking action and constantly grinding.

The problem was that he constantly waited to take action, which made sure that he constantly doubted himself. You can't doubt yourself while you're performing an action. You either try or you don't. That's it. So learn to take action because a magical fairy with her confidence dust won't be coming anytime soon. She won't sprinkle that shit on you.

You just have to keep on taking action and keep moving forward. There's no time to doubt yourself if you're in motion. Remember that line because it makes a huge difference!

300. SINGLE AND ASSUMING TO BE READY TO MINGLE

S o many people are unhappily single, but they fall into a trap here. They can't make themselves happy and they assume that someone else will do it. But how can you make another person happy if you can't make yourself happy? I mean, how does that even work? Do you really think that you can love somebody else if you can't love yourself? That's the most ridiculous thing that I've ever heard and yes, I'm aware that some people claim that the Earth to be flat.

Understand that you can never make another person happy and that nobody can make you happy. You're happy from within or you're not. There's no middle grounjd here. So you are either desperate or you're not. It's really that simple.

301. I LIVE IN THE NOW, LEARN FROM THE PAST AND WORK FOR THE FUTURE

Most people live in the past because they want to change it. They also neglect the now, so they miss out on all the opportunities in front of them. Instead, they dream about the future.

I don't regret past events because I always learn a lesson which ensures that I can move on. I live in the now because I want to be aware of the opportunities that are right in front of me. Nobody wants to miss out on those.

I also work for a better future. Most people dream about a better future, but they waste a lot of time while they dream. So they never get anything done and the dream eventually turns into a complete nightmare. You need to be aware of the past, present and future. Mixing these up might ruin your whole life.

302. POLITICIANS ARE HIGH-PAID CLOWNS WHO WEAR EXPENSIVES SUIT INSTEAD RED NOSES

I posted this online on the day that we had to vote here in Belgium. Politicians are the only people who can answer a simple "yes" and "no" question with a three-hour answer. Sometimes it amazes me, to be honest.

To add to that, I don't really get why people like to involve themselves in politics so much since these people always end up disappointed with them. Don't focus too much on politics unless you really want to have a career in politics. It won't make you a better person and it won't bring you closer to your goals, so why even bother?

303. REVENGE HURTS THE OTHER PERSON ONCE WHILE IT HURTS YOU TWICE

Some people really like to take vengeance, but they don't get that it hurts them twice.

Let me explain. I once hit my old trainer's eye with my knee in grappling. It was a dumb accident, but he decided to manhandle me in response. He could have really hurt me, but he didn't care. It wasn't the first time that he had done something like that; he even injured one of my training partners because he was eagerly looking for vengeance.

We had to shake hands, of course, when training was done and he looked down at the floor when we shook. He was really embarrassed for his actions, I think.

This was yet another reason why I left that gym. Looking for vengeance usually makes things a lot worse and it makes sure that you lose, too. It hurts the other person once, but it'll hurt you twice.

304. PEOPLE CLAIM THAT THE SKY IS THE LIMIT, BUT WE'VE BEEN ON THE MOON

This was a social media post that I came up with after someone claimed that the sky is the limit. That would have been true if we hadn't been on the moon already. Now we're going to be on Mars a few years from now. Do you get where I'm going with this?

People always claim that they can't do things that've already been achieved. Seriously - stop putting limits on yourself. Just start doing things and try to forget about limits. They're called "limits" because they'll limit you. You have no clue how much potential you've got and I'm pretty sure that nobody ever comes close to his real potential.

305. PEOPLE WHO HATE THEIR MORNINGS HATE THEIR LIVES

There are people who get up and life feels like a struggle to them. They hate everything and everyone. How can you have a great day if you don't kickstart it in the morning?

Understand that you will never get the perfect morning, but you really end up hating your life if you hate your mornings. How can you hate the morning if you haven't even done anything yet? It means that you really aren't looking forward to the rest of the day, so it's safe to assume that you really don't like your life.

So why not make a change. Why don't you make sure that you really look forward to getting up. The only reason that I sleep is because I get the value of sleep. I really don't hate my mornings because I mostly start the day with something that I really like.

306. THE TRUTH HURTS YOU IN THE SHORT TERM WHILE LIES HURT YOU IN THE LONG TERM. PICK YOUR POISON.

Most people are hurt when they hear the truth, but the truth can make sure that you actually grow in an area of which you weren't aware previously. Still, so many people decide to tell other people lies to comfort them, so these people start to believe these things. This just hurts them big time in the long run because they keep on living lives based on these lies.

It's not comfortable to tell people the truth, but it's better to be a good friend and tell the truth than to lie because it also hurts you in the long run. People will be mad at you because you've sold them lies. So you're either an asshole in the immediate future or an asshole later on. Pick your poison, I guess. You'll have to pick one either way.

307. YOU ARE WHAT YOU REPEATEDLY DO, SO DON'T DO USELESS STUFF

This is from a Greek philosopher and he's right. You really are what you repeatedly do, so don't do useless stuff because you'll end up being useless.

So many people get caught up in doing useless stuff. I don't know anybody who's not prone to it. We all tend to spend way too much time on social media. But we can change this habit and do something a lot better and more productive. So try to read a book instead of spending time on social media. Cuddle with your girlfriend instead of staring at your phone first thing in the morning. Just replace a bad habit with a good one and you'll change your life in no time!

We are what we repeatedly do, so let's be useful instead of useless.

308. "NO" MEANS NO AND "YES" MEANS YES

People seem to misunderstand this, but it's so simple. "No" means no and "yes" means yes. People who don't understand this are just playing an act. Of course they understand this, but they don't like the outcome, so they start to ask questions to make sure that they can change the outcome.

Don't even bother defending yourself with these kind of people. They understood from the start and they played stupid in order to manipulate you. I even know people who'll try to make me feel guilty when I say no to them. Weird but true.

309. NEVER BITE A HELPING HAND

I t was raining on a Saturday and my grandmother needed a lift to be able to do her groceries because she doesn't have a driver's license. So she called me to ask if I could pick her up and help her. I told her that that was fine, but we had to do it at three in the afternoon because I had a training session at five.

At first, she said that she was only available at 5:00 and that she couldn't do groceries earlier, so I was like, "OK, so then I can't help you today." She quickly realized that she couldn't pull her tricks with me and suddenly "remembered" that she would be available sooner in the day.

People are always complaining when someone offers them help. I quickly made my grandmother realize that I wanted to help her, but that I didn't want to skip training. She got what she need and I didn't have to skip training. Two people were made happy that day.

310. BE OPEN-MINDED AND CLOSE-MINDED AT THE SAME TIME

People always say that you should be open-minded, but this is pretty dangerous if you ask me. I've noticed that open-minded people are prone to being distracted so damn easily. They're too open-minded.

Being close-minded and open-minded at the same time means that you don't give in to distractions. I mean, doing coke and hookers all weekend sounds like a lot of fun to some people, but it won't do me any good. Reading a book about human behavior might help me in life.

It's about constantly trying to find a balance and trying to realize what's important and what isn't. Some things should be left alone so find balance in your mindset and learn to be less curious to things that don't benefit you at all.

311. ONLY PEOPLE WHO READ BETWEEN THE LINES WILL BE COMPLETELY FINE

E ver noticed that you can't understand stuff from some self-help books or even the Bible unless you read between the lines? People want to be given directions directly, but smart people tend to speak in riddles from time to time. They don't get that not everything should be interpreted literally.

This is the fault of the educational system, in my opinion. They just make you repeat so many things that you lose track of how you can progress. It's by reading between the lines.

Read *Think And Grow Rich* to see if you're able to understand it. That book should be read between the lines. My dad claims that it's complete garbage, while I claim that it's a masterpiece. Guess who can't read between the lines.

312. YOUR MIND IS LIKE A PARACHUTE. YOU'RE IN TROUBLE WHEN IT'S NOT OPEN.

You need to have an open mind to be able to progress in life. People with a closed mind can't learn anything because they claim that they know it all. These so-called experts mostly learn nothing new because they just don't want to. Be aware of this mindset flaw. The only way to be sure that you're not closed-minded is to actually question the fact that you're close-minded. People who're close minded will usually say that they're not.

So your mind should be like a parachute. It only benefits you when it's open. Do I need to say more? I seriously hope that I don't have to!

313. YOU CAN'T POUR MORE WATER IN A CUP THAT'S ALREADY FULL

This principle applies to the open/closed mind debate. People who're closed-minded are like a cup that's full. You can't add anything and they probably wouldn't let you either.

I shared a lot of things with people when I started my self-development journey. I quickly realized that they mostly didn't even cared or even laughed at what I said. The cup was full and pouring over. It's weird, but some people just don't like to learn new things in life. So empty your cup and try to fill it up with other people's knowledge. You really don't want to become dumber and dumber, do you?

314. EVERY GREAT STORY STARTS WITH FAILURE OR ADVERSITY NOT WITH VODKA

People always claim that the best stories start with alcohol. I get where it comes from. We all have some fun stories from the times when we were drunk, but they're not the best stories. My story and a lot of other people's stories started off with pain, struggle and the fact that we all hit rock bottom. We all built ourselves up from that point.

Now that's a really great story. There's not a single drunk story in my life that made people go, "wow, you really turned your life around." It entertains them, but you can entertain people without alcohol, so why would you even bother getting drunk all the time? Turn your life around and make yourself proud.

315. YOU'RE A PRODUCT OF YOUR ACTIONS, NOT YOUR FEELINGS

People don't get that you aren't a product of your feelings. Wel,1 you are and aren't. Say, for example, that you've got to fight in a cage. You're going to be afraid, right? I mean, who wouldn't? But the feeling doesn't determine who you are because everybody is afraid. What determines who you are is how you deal with that feeling. You either give in completely or you're brave and actually go out and fight.

People don't see how you feel, they just see how you act and they'll put a label on you based on that. So always take the hard road in life. It'll make you a lot tougher.

316. "DREAM, BELIEVE, ACHIEVE" DOESN'T WORK

I really like the book *Think And Grow Rich,* but one of the main ideas from the book is that you should "dream, believe, achieve." This might work for some people, but it doesn't turn out so great for most people. They mostly dream, believe and never achieve.

That sounds pretty disappointing, doesn't it? So what's the alternative? "Plan, work, believe, achieve." Seriously, that's how it works. It doesn't sound pretty, but the reality isn't like it's portrayed in the movies. You better not neglect the "work" part because otherwise you'll never achieve.

So why don't you try plan, work, believe, achieve instead of dream, believe, achieve? It might actually benefit you in the long run.

317. THE PROBLEM IS THAT YOU ASSUME YOU'VE GOT TIME WHILE TIME IT'S ACTUALLY RUNNING OUT

I'll never forget this lesson. It was on an off day and I had just woken up. I felt a little bit lazy and assumed that I still had a lot of time left in the day, but then I realized that time was actually running out. This made a huge impact on me. I soon realized that this is applicable to life as well.

We all have dreams and goals which we put on the backburner because we've got time, but do we really have time or is it just running out? I assume that the second answer is more fitting when it comes to life. The "time" concept is a dangerous one. It's good to be optimistic, but it's also important to be realistic.

318. YOU CAN BE WEALTHY YET COMPLETELY POOR. YOU CAN BE POOR YET EXTREMELY WEALTHY.

C an you guess to what I'm referring to here? I'm refer-ring to happiness. People want to be rich, but I've never heard someone claim that they wanted to be happy. Well, I have, but they're the minority of the population.

I've seen people who barely had anything who were so ex-tremely happy. I assume that it was because they were more grateful for everything they got. That's something that most rich people or people in general miss out on. They assume that money can buy happiness, but it can't. You'll just feel empty down the line without understanding why. Money can't buy happiness. It's crazy that people don't see this by now.

319. PROGRESS BEATS PAIN

I'll never forget the first time that I got hit with a liver shot in sparring. It hurts a lot; your body completely shuts down. But can you guess what happened the next sparring when the guy tried it again? My defense was in place. He was only able to catch me once more with it over a period of two years.

When he caught me, it was after a month layoff and I was completely gassed, but even then I learned a lesson. So what's the lesson here? We all face points in life where we're hurt. This can be mentally or physically, but you can't beat this pain by complaining. You just need to make progress and then you'll get rid of the pain. "No pain, no gain" is a saying for a reason.

320. FIND YOUR "WHY" AND THE "HOW" WILL TAKE CARE OF ITSELF

I almost quit MMA at one point because I was sick of training at my old gym. I was so close of pulling the plug until I heard this one simple question on a podcast: "Why did you start?"

I had completely lost sight of why I had started in the first place, to be honest. I was so caught up in the emotions that I didn't focus on the "why." I eventually found my why again when someone advised me to check out the gym at which I'm currently training. I checked it out and was sold right away.

People lose a lot of time figuring out how they're going to achieve something and that's important, too. But you're going to break if you don't find your why. You why is what keeps you going. It's the light in the dark. The how is constantly changing and less important than the why.

321. PEOPLE WOULD RATHER GOOGLE AN EXCUSE THAN ACTUALLY PUT IN THE WORK

I've got a lot of opinions on this matter, but this quote sums my feelings up very well. I like it the most because it's close to reality. So many people claim that they want something out of life, but they put more work in looking for excuses than actually getting results.

It's pretty amazing, right? The fact that some people actually want to put in more work in sabotaging themselves really makes me wonder how we've gotten that far. I mean, why would you sabotage your own potential? Please don't try to google the answer. There are already more than enough dumb questions asked on Google.

322. CHEAP SHOTS FROM A CHEAP GUY

I often buy cigars for two buddies of mine. They normally pay me back, but one of them still owes me some money. He knows this because he has since rejected my offers to bring a cigar for him when we pla on smoking.

This changed when we had a party at a friend's house. The couple had some expensive cigars which they had bought in Cuba. The guy who still owes me money was offered one and refused, but then he asked from whom they were. He picked the most expensive of all the cigars when he knew that they weren't mine and that they were free.

This was a disgusting act, in my opinion. How low can you go? Pretty low apparently. Oh, we aren't buddies anymore either, but I guess that this isn't a surprise to you.

323. WRITING THIS BOOK WAS NOT THAT HARD

Weird, right? I've never written such a huge amount in such a short period of time, but somehow I managed to pull it off.

Do you want to know my secret? It's pretty simple. I mostly sit back quietly and observe my environment. Just take a look at how many of these chapters are related to my personal life. I learned a lot from observing or talking to other people. All those lessons were learned over the course of a little more than two years. I decided to put them into a book to make sure that I would never forget them and I realized that they could benefit other people as well.

324. INSTANT GRATIFICATION LEADS TO LONG-TERM FRUSTRATION

This is applicable to almost everything in life. Fast doesn't equal good. Things that come easily are mostly cursed, but I get that you want them because you want results and you want them fast.

You want to bang that hot girl, but you don't want to get to know her, so you're surprised when she turns out to be a total bitch.

You want to be filthy rich, but you don't want to work, so you play the lottery. You're hoping to win the big prize while you know deep down inside that you're going to be broke again.

There are tons of examples, but the main principle is easy to understand: instant gratification leads to long-term frustration. So be smart and avoid a bad start. It might be sunshine and rainbows in the beginning, but the sun doesn't shine 24/7. Welcome to the real life.

325. I CAN'T RELATE TO LAZY PEOPLE, BUT I DON'T WANT TO EITHER

L azy people are one of a kind, I've got to give them that. But I don't get that they can live like this. We speak completely different languages. I seriously don't get how people can waste so much time doing nothing. Those people are bored all the time. It's literally a miracle that they can't find anything useful to do with heir time. You can literally learn almost anything from YouTube these days, but you can also find a lot of dumb shit on there.

Lazy people are on a constant quest to stay in their comfort zones. It's really weird that those people prefer to stay in bed instead of actually doing something useful. They're basically like little kids that have no clue what to do and then starts to complain when they feel bored.

I don't understand, but I don't want to understand either, to be honest. I just like to focus on getting things done. They claim that I'm crazy while I say that they're lazy.

326. KARMA MIGHT BE A BITCH, BUT SO ARE YOU

There's something odd that I noticed recently. A lot of people are claiming that othersare extremely rude. These people have only gotten one part of the equation. They get that others should be nice, but they don't live by their own rule. So these people act rude and act surprised when they don't get away with it.

Every action has a reaction. So these people suddenly act like victims. They try to make other people feel guilty. What a bitch move. They just project how they feel onto you. These people lose friends all the time and don't get why. I get it.

327. LET'S TALK ABOUT SEX, BABY, LET'S TALK ABOUT YOU - NOT ME (PART I)

I know that this book is full of examples from my own life, but this chapter will be an exception. You see, I've never fucked around like most guys do. It's a waste of time that will leave you with nothing but an empty feeling and frustration.

Most guys fuck around to serve their ego (the "bro, I fucked two girls this week!" guy). My friend, I really don't care. I'm not impressed by how many girls you've fucked. You might impress a lot of people, but I'm just not one of them. I don't follow the herd. I have an own opinion and I'm not afraid to share it. I wouldn't change my reaction to boost your ego either. Your fragile ego leaves me cold. These guys' whole image is based on how successful they are with girls. So they feel like an alpha because they're able to score all the time.

328. LET'S TALK ABOUT SEX, BABY, LET'S TALK ABOUT YOU - NOT ME (PART II)

There are just two problems when it comes to this matter.

First, these guys' egos are extremely fragile because they're actually insecure. They just don't want to show it to the world. Alpha males don't have fragile egos, so I guess that you're not as tough as you imagined.

The second problem is that they attract wounded animals with their whole act. Pick-up artists are great in teaching guys how to act like an alpha. They practice scenarios and it works. But it'll only work on the drama queens or the ones that can't see through your act. A classy girl will smell the act from a mile away and just tell you to go away.

329. UNMOTIVATED? THIS ONE EASY TRICK IS GOING TO HELP.

I never feel unmotivated to train MMA, so that's easy. But I sometimes feel unmotivated to write blog posts. It's hard from time to time since I sometimes can't seem to find a topic to write about. Don't forget that I've released four posts a week since October 2016. That's a pretty long time.

But I'm not here to makes excuses, I'm here to help you! My trick is applicable to everything, by the way. I sit in front of my computer and just tell myself that I'm going to write one sentence. After that, I see how I feel. I'm allowed to quit here, but I'm long-gone at this point. I keep on writing until I've got a blog. It's pretty funny that I can trick myself over and over again.

I assume that I'm just not prone to laziness. I really hate doing nothing. So to all the people who feel unmotivated to work out, don't fall into the trap you lay down for yourself after you come home from work. Don't start to watch television. Drink some water, eat some honey and do some push-ups. You'll suddenly feel better and keep on going. The mind is such a beautiful thing if you know how to use it.

330. UNMOTIVATED? WATCH OUT FOR THIS.

Your body could be in a state of overtraining. Then it becomes dangerous to push yourself. People who are overtrained feel unmotivated as well. Those people should take one or even two weeks off. (Don't worry - you can't be overtrained if you never train.)

People who are overtrained mostly get injured before they even notice that they're overtraining. So learn the difference between being overtrained and being unmotivated.

A simple trick is to monitor your heart rate first thing in the morning. Mine is usually below 50 or slightly above it. You should take a day off if your heartbeat is 10 beats per minute higher than normal. I took another day off yesterday because I knew that training was a bad idea. It's all about listening to your body.

331. COLLEGE LIFE IS EXTREMELY OVERRATED

Many people love their time in college so much because they had so much freedom. You're basically allowed to do whatever you want. I've seen guys go out at night and come drunk to class the next day because they hadn't slept. Those people act are pretty happy in their comfort zone.

But after college, they get a real job, a "serious" relationship and so on. They suddenly feel stuck and constantly look back at the past, which is depressing. They're not craving the college life; they're craving freedom. They just don't realize it yet.

Those people want to act like there is no limit. They want to ball like most rappers and bang like Hugh Hefner. Those guys are clearly facing midlife crises, which is extremely stupid if you ask me. I'd rather still be married by the time I reach the age where I could have a midlife crisis.

332. COLLEGE LIFE & THE INEVITABLE MIDLIFE CRISIS

People who are facing a midlife crisis act really dumb. They basically act like little boys. They cheat on their wives, buy a motorcycle and so on. Can you guess how it ends? They regret it all.

Your actions have consequences, so you'd better think things through. People who face midlife crises often just realize that they're mortal and they haven't lived to their full potential. The strange thing is that they degrade themselves instead of living up to their full potential. Well, it's not weird because that's the easy way out. That's probably something they've done a thousand times over the years, so it became a habit.

Well, I don't have proof that I'm right, so this is just a theory. I've never heard of people who have faced midlife crises and truly lived up to their potential. So I might be wrong on this one, but I might be right as well. It's up to you to decide if you like the theory or not.

333. COLLEGE LIFE: USE YOUR TIME WISELY

You'll never have as much free time as you have in college, so why don't you use it wisely? I used it wisely in my last year (before the inevitable dropout). Work on something that you really want to do (like a blog) or learn something new. You can still party from time to time. Moderation is the key here.

I started this blog when I was in college and I planned my way out. I skipped basically every single class and made the most of my time. So you can do the same, but don't skip classes so that you get your degree if you really want to achieve it.

Oh, and one more thing: don't chase girls. It's tempting to do this when you're in college, but the guys who do it are miserable later on in life. I recently saw one of those cool kids from college. He was completely out of shape and had no clue on how to spend his time. Only a fool chases everything that's cool.

334. THE BEST MOTIVATIONAL SPEECH THAT I EVER HEARD (PART I)

L et's talk about the best motivational speech that I ever heard. A lot of people are big fans of motivational speeches these days. The speeches fire them up, but they all wait for the perfect moment to use this energy. There's no such thing as the perfect Monday, but keep on looking. You'll just find frustration and misery if you're taking that road.

But I guess that you're here to find out which motivational speech is the best? Or at least the best in my opinion? It's not a long one. The speech contained two simple words. These two words really lit a fire inside of me. The person who said this to me spoke only two words:

"YOU CAN'T."

335. THE BEST MOTIVATIONAL SPEECH THAT I'VE EVER HEARD (PART II)

Man, I laughed so hard when this guy told me this. This guy was just projecting his own insecurities onto me. That's what most insecure people do. They want to keep others down on their own level. So they discourage others from improving themselves.

Dream killers are egocentric people and they don't even realize it. I don't waste a lot of time on these people. Those people become dumber over time and they can't improve because there's something blocking their own potential. It's their own ego.

Stupidity + ego = a dangerous cocktail without self-improvement.

336. ISN'T THAT THE BEST MOTIVATIONAL SPEECH YOU'VE EVER HEARD?

Some people will claim that it's far from the best motivational speech that they've ever heard and I get why. Some people really get discouraged when they hear that they shouldn't try something. But that's just stupid because you're deciding to stop pursuing something which you really like. You stop because your opinion is based on that of others and that's pretty damn sad.

I've got one simple question for you: who's going to believe in you if you don't even believe in yourself? Nobody! So learn to master the art of not giving a fuck and turn the "I can't" into an "I can"!

337. NEW YEAR RESOLUTIONS ARE FOR DRUNK PEOPLE (PART I)

Do you tend to make new year resolutions? I advise you to invest your time in something else if you answered yes. You're wasting precious time and you know it. You're just too lazy to act upon this feeling. New year resolutions are for the drunk and the miserable.

I seriously don't even get why people those resolutions anyway. Well, I actually do get it. People have drunk personalities and seem to get that they're not so happy after all. So they make up some New Year's resolutions which they eventually forget the next day due to a hangover. I mean, there are people who have been claiming that they'll take up a sport since 2013. I sometimes wonder if they still believe it after so many years.

Most people even laugh at their own resolutions while they're making them. They say stuff like, "I'll resolve to accomplish the same things as last year since I didn't accomplish any of them."

It's never too late to change, of course. Just don't make ew year resolutions; those are a real waste of time.

338. NEW YEAR'S RESOLUTIONS ARE FOR DRUNK PEOPLE (PART II)

So I guess that you realize I'm not a big believer in those resolutions. Can you guess why? Because most people just make claims like that all the time without ever putting a date on it. Those resolutions are vague and will never turn into reality.

Can you guess where we're heading? It's time to set goals. Goal setting is a lot better because you put a date to something. For example, "I want to be in shape by 01/06/2019." Now you've got something to work with. The guy that makes a resolution to be in shape one day will never be in shape.

I use this technique all the time. I take a notebook and write down my goals in the same fashion ("I want to achieve X before Y."). That's goal setting to the max. Just make sure that you make realistic goals. You can't get in shape in a single day and you won't be able to buy your dream car by next week without going broke.

339. SO WHAT'S YOUR RECAP OF YOUR YEAR? LET'S FIND OUT.

Most people never recap their year because they assume that they're going to live forever. They literally deny their own mortality. That's really sad if you ask me.

Now I'm going to ask you a simple question and, in most cases, I think I will know the answer. How many goals did you have this year and how many goals did you accomplish? You can't accomplish things if you don't set goals.

The second question isn't an easy one either: how did you improve this year? Most people's highlights of the year are the times where they didn't have to work or where they could party all night long. They usually don't remember the latter and were bored to death when they didn't work.

So where does this leave us? What's the summary of your year? Has anything even changed at all? I advise you to be brutally honest with yourself and change for the better if you answered "no" to my last question. My friend, the day that you stop learning is the day that you start dying. Remember that.

340. LOOKS AREN'T EVERYTHING IN LIFE

This might be one of the shocking of my life lessons, but I mean it. I have a cauliflower ear (google it if you don't know what it is) due to grappling. I also have a black eye at this time. So people have been staring at me because I look like I had been involved in a fist fight.

I still have a particular quote in mind when people start to point out my ear:

A wise man once said: "beauty is the worst trait that you can own."

You're nothing with beauty on its own. What if a beautiful girl acts like a complete bitch? I wouldn't date her. I wouldn't date a dumb girl who's pretty either. Most guys would do it, but I wouldn't. I'd rather be with an average girl who is a catch than a 10/10 girl who's dumb and arrogant. I would ditch the latter for sure. You need more than fancy looks to impress me.

Just be yourself because that's a challenge on its own.

341. NEVER KISS ON THE FIRST DATE

Y ou should never kiss because it's a recipe for disaster. Most people want to go way too fast. They want instant gratification but end up with long-term frustration.

Why do people kiss on the first date anyway? Because all your friends tell you that you should? Maybe because you don't want to be lonely? You should aim for a solid base first before you move on to the next level. So it's best to be sure that you know the other person well before you move on to the next level.

You might assume that I'm a bit boring, but I have one simple message for you. My life isn't a reality TV show. You can draw your own conclusions.

Take it slow. That's what smart people do.

342. YOU SEE THE POTENTIAL IN A PERSON WHEN YOU DATE

I dated a girl earlier this year and I assumed that we would have tons of dates. It didn't turn out the way that I thought it would be. She was a different person when we met the second time. I didn't understand this until someone told me that you always see the potential in the people you date. It all made sense after that.

That's another reason why you shouldn't kiss on the first date. People will eventually show their true nature. They either live up to the potential or they don't. Some people want to grow while others will hold you down. So it's better to wait and see if people truly live up to their potential. Most people, sadly, don't.

343. PEOPLE LIKE TO BE LONELY TOGETHER

People can't be alone. They just can't. I realized this when I went to a restaurant on my own. People were giving me weird looks since I was there by myself. I gave those people a topic to talk about, to be honest. Soon, they all returned to staring mode. They just sat in front of each other in silence. So I either go with real friends or I go on my own.

The same goes for relationships. People don't care about who they date. They just want to be with someone so that they aren't alone. It's extremely pathetic if you can't be alone. Grow up! Be with someone that you really like or learn to be alone. Don't act like a little kid. You'll never be able to make a person happy if you're not able to make yourself happy. Remember that you're in really bad company if you start feeling alone.

344. FRIENDS? EVERYBODY IS REPLACEABLE.

This may sound harsh, but I stand by my opinion. I don't care about looks, how long I've know certain people, if they're family or not, and so on. You're replaceable if you know me. I follow the "two strikes and you're out" approach.

I can guarantee you that a lot of people assumed that I was kidding about that, but I wasn't. Those people aren't a part of my life anymore and they probably still don't get why. The reason is pretty simple: you tried to screw me more than once and now you're out. Or you disappointed me twice and you're out.

Life's too short to spend time with people who are not worth it. This approach makes life so much easier.

345. HARD WORK PAYS OFF IN THE LONG RUN

You can have all the talent in the world, but you won't outwork me. You're competing with the wrong guy when it comes to that matter. Here's a story to prove it.

I trained at All-Stars MMA in the summer of 2017, the gym of Alexander "The Mauler" Gustafsson. We did a hard conditioning workout that lasted an hour. We were all drenched in sweat when the workout was over. I was preparing to do some extra work, but no one else was up for it. So I was doing my thing and they all left because they were tired. All but one guy.

I had noticed that he kept on watching me because he wanted to see when I was going to quit. He eventually left after an hour and I trained for another hour after that. You see, I didn't compete with him. I competed with myself. That guy quit because he was trying to compete with me.

Winners focus on winning while losers focus on winners. Remember that quote.

346. DO WHAT YOU LOVE TO GET RID OF FEAR

Have you ever tried something new but eventually quit because somebody mocked you? I was mocked once on Facebook by a girl who was citing part of a blog post. I just "liked" her comment.

People like to mock others all the time. You've got to do something that you really like in order to make sure that you don't stop when people hate on you. That's the secret. Well, not really a secret, but most people don't get it. They shy away from things because they're afraid of the hate.

I didn't care about her comment and you know why? Because I love blogging, plus it says a lot about her as well. She was giving me free advertising because people became curious about my blog after reading her comment.

There's no point in taking the hateful comments seriously. I mean, who even makes time to hate on others? (Bonus point for you if you said "miserable people.")

347. THERE'S ALWAYS A SOLUTION BUT NEVER A PROBLEM

I still have a couple of life lessons left. Isn't it crazy that I learned so much over the course of a couple of yeas? It just made me smile for a minute.

People tend to focus way too much on the problem and that's why they can't solve it. I, on the other hand, focus on the solution and always fix it. That's why most people shy away from failure while I embrace it.

I once broke my nose (well, it was heavily bruised, anyway) in a sparring session. My nose kept on bleeding for 15 minutes. Most people would quit here,but I just wanted to know what I did wrong and get back on the mats. I was out for a week, but the experience didn't hold me back.

I found the solution to the problem and it won't happen again. Lesson learned. Next, please!

348. SLOW PROGRESS IS PROGRESS

People aren't patient when it comes to certain things. They all want them as soon as possible. People focus on the outcome instead of the process. I focus on the process instead of the outcome. I love the process. It's the most beautiful thing there is.

There are times, though, where the process gets frustrating because you don't seem to progress at all, but you've got to keep trying. Suddenly, you'll see progress and keep on progressing. The end result is fun for maybe three seconds, but the process doesn't bore me at all. Time flies by and that's when you're focusing on the process.

In conclusion: don't stop because your progress is a bit slower than usual. Keep going and eventually your progress will skyrocket. Nobody knows how long it'll take. It takes as long as it takes. The worst thing you could do is being impatient.

349. NEED A PURPOSE TO BE HAPPY IN LIFE

You need a goal, a purpose or just something bigger than yourself to get up first thing in the morning. People assume that I perform some kind of magic trick when I get up first thing in the morning. In reality, I don't. I have a purpose in life and that's the reason why I don't waste time.

I look forward to the weekends because I've got even more time to be productive. Other people hate the weekends because they've got so much spare time. So these people party until they pass out from all the booze they've indulged.

People perform all kinds of escapism just to avoid a reality check. Face it: you've got no clue what you want in life, so everything that kills time is perfect in your opinion. Just ask yourself the following question: are you really happy sleeping until noon on the weekends? Or are you really happy when you chase girls? The answer is no. You're just bored and I don't how you can be bored in this day and age.

350. DO YOU WORK TO LIVE OR LIVE TO WORK?

D o you work to live or live to work? Now that's a hard question, isn't it? This was said by a guy in BJJ after a pretty hard sparring session. I forgot how we ended up talking about this topic.

It's a great question if you ask me since most people don't think about it. These people just drift through life. They go with the flow as they like to say, but they have no clue where they're heading. That's what you get when you've got no sense of purpose in life. You'll basically end up anywhere. It means that you could gain a promotion or a burnout. The odds are even and you don't know what you'll get.

I seriously hope that you won't face a burnout. It mostly goes downhill from there for most people. That's what happens if you live to work.

351. EVERYTHING I DO WON'T BE FOR YOU.

People give up all their dreams when they meet someone new. Can you guess the major flaw in your relationship approach? It's pretty easy if you ask me:

NEVER EVER CHANGE YOURSELF FOR A WOMAN.

She was attracted to you with a reason and you're taking it away. You're going to lose your relationship if you put your hobbies or ambitions aside for her. I made this mistake myself. I don't regret the fact that I stopped playing soccer, but the reason why I did it was stupid. I eventually found MMA, so I can't complain.

I learned this lesson later on, but I was mad at myself as I became single. I really wished that I hadn't given up on soccer at that time. You can call your girlfriend "the one" if you want, but you have to act like a man and never put your own needs on the backburner. You'll lose precious time and she's not worth the time if she doesn't support you. Remember that it can be extremely dangerous for your mental health if you stay in a toxic relationship.

352. ARE YOU FEELING SAD AND LONELY ON VALENTINE'S DAY?

Are you feeling sad and lonely on Valentine's day? Man, that must be a bummer, but I'm not a part of that group even though I am single and have been for a long time. It must have been about four years now.

I had this problem as well in the past, but then I realized that I was the one who created it. So I solved it, but that's what most people don't do. They can't be alone and that's the start of a lot of problems.

There's another big problem and that's that their ego can't handle the fact that they're alone. They don't get why they're single. Let me put it this way: ego is the anesthesia that deadens the pain of stupidity. You won't get a lot out of life if you've got a giant ego. Anyway, think about Valentine's Day and why it shouldn't affect your mood: it's just a day like any other! That's it!

353. PAIN IS CRUEL, BUT YOU CAN USE IT AS FUEL.

When you're in a state of pain, there are two ways to look at it. You can either let break you down or lift you up.

Pain can actually motivate you to become a better version of yourself. Without my depression, I never would have become the guy I am today. Such events motivate me to do better than I did prior to them. The events actually got me back on track as soon as I understood them and got rid of the pain.

People don't realize this, but the lesson here is that the cure of the pain is always in the pain itself. The only thing that you need to do is accept the pain and that's the hardest part. It's hard to accept pain because it's a horrible feeling. But you can't be happy if you're never sad. Life's all about balance.

354. SO TELL ME, DO YOU COUNT ON FAITH TO SOLVE THINGS?

I like having a mentor. (I felt this way even before I took on Sean Fagan as my mentor). I've had multiple mentors, actually. You see, when I dropped out of college, I made a huge goal list and getting a mentor was a top priority. It's easier to learn from others' mistakes because sometimes they make you see things in another way.

That's what happened. We were talking about my future goals, failures and faith. I told him that I plan to keep working towards my goals and that faith would take care of the rest. I literally said this: "I can't fail because I've got faith on my side."

He then told me something pretty remarkable. He told me that I had confidence in myself but that I wasn't acknowledging it. So I reflected on this and then it struck me. All the things that suggested faith was helping me out were just the result of the fact that I took action and was not willing to give in. I'm still pretty spiritual but am aware that believing in faith can make people pretty passive.

355. HOW CAN YOU LIVE IF YOU NEVER CHALLENGE YOUR BELIEFS?

L et's take a look at some popular beliefs:

"You need to have a degree and work until the age 65."

"Always kiss at the end of the first or second date. Otherwise, you'll end up in the friend zone."

"Being single for a long time is unacceptable."

"People who don't have a degree are losers."

"You have to watch the news in order to be smart."(Read this blog because that's not true.)

The list goes on and on.

But who claims that those things are true? Just think about it. Is there actual proof that these things are 100% true? Most people can't answer this question, but they're afraid to challenge their own beliefs.

356. WHY I ACTUALLY DISLIKE THE TERM "ALPHA MALE"

A friend of mine called me "Mr. Alpha" once. I liked the name, so I stuck with it as a joke. You see, I don't like the term because so many guys use it to their own advantage. Most guys just act really dumb and still claim to be alpha. Many people seem to approve of it as well. Then you hear stuff like, "that guy is really big and scores women all the time. He's the real deal. He's an alpha."

There's nothing alpha about being big and there's nothing alpha about scoring women all the time. Guys who act like this have almost nothing to offer. I challenge you to talk with those guys about how they feel. None of them will be able to do it. They'll laugh at you, mock you ("You're not a pussy, are you?") or just avoid your questions altogether.

It's an act and it's an act that doesn't lead to happiness in life. Those people are mostly extremely unhappy and unfulfilled. These are the ones who do all kinds of crazy stuff just out of unhappiness. Stuff like drugs, excessive alcohol, chasing women, and worse.

357. HONESTY IS A VERY EXPENSIVE GIFT.

Honesty is a very expensive gift, so don't expect it from cheap people. There are a lot of people who don't like me, but can you guess why? Because I'm not afraid of telling the truth and nobody likes to hear the truth. Because the truth shows you things about yourself that you didn't want to acknowledge yet or that you will never acknowledge at all.

It's like the time when I realized that I was going bald. I did a lot to hide it like most guys but eventually, I just shaved it off. You can't escape the truth forever or you'll just live in an imaginary world where everybody but you knows that you're lying.

Honesty is a virtue which I highly value. The same goes for respect and integrity. There are more virtues which are important but most people can't even fit those, so why even mention the rest?

358. WRITE, BECAUSE IT HEALS THE SOUL AND RELAXES THE MIND.

D id you know that I write every single day? I blog (or I journal because I don't share everything on my blog). I can't share everything - that would be stupid. So I only share the things which could help other people to improve their lives.

I always write on my own. There's never somebody around when I do it. I basically use the power of silence and solitude to my advantage. You need to be focused when you do it.

So let's assume that you're facing a problem. Why don't you write about it? I can assure you that you could end up with pages about a certain issue. Write about the problems and write about how you feel. You should even try to see the issue from the other person's perspective.

359. WHY YOU SHOULD CALL PEOPLE OUT ON THEIR BULLSHIT

So why should you call people out their own lies? Well, because nobody gets better by it. You've got nothing to gain from lies from another person, but that person won't gain anything as well. You didn't hear the truth, but the other person didn't tell the truth, so in the end, you'll be both miserable. That sucks.

So call them out. It might be uncomfortable and they might call you a jerk, but look at it from another perspective. Who is actually the jerk here? The one that lies or the one that calls the liar out?

You're basically offering those people an opportunity to grow here. How can you be a jerk if you make people better? Well, that's easy. Because nobody like to hear the truth. Nobody wants to hear that they're underperforming on their own potential. There would be a lot less cheating in this world if people were more honest. People prefer to be unhappy instead of hearing the truth.

360. THE WORD "ADULT" MEANS ABSOLUTELY NOTHING

Remember when you turned 18? You finally turned into an adult. Suddenly, you were allowed to sit at the big table to talk about serious things. Life was about to start and you felt like the man.

Well, you felt like that until you finally spent some time with those adults. They weren't as mature as you first thought they would be. They haven't much too talked about anything at all and their actions are far from adulthood worthy.

This is sad, right? I mean, their egos get bigger and bigger, but their thinking capability diminishes. That's something that I've seen with a lot of people. The word "adult" means absolutely nothing. It's a hollow word and here's why.

361. MOST ADULTS ARE ARROGANT AND QUESTION NOTHING

Ever seen a little kid question something that an adult said? Ever seen how angry the adult gets when they're suddenly in a position in which they would lose an argument against a little kid or just someone younger? They get angry because their egos can't handle it. So try to win the argument by telling the other person that they should listen to them because they're the adult.

I have one simple message for these people. Age is just a number and doesn't reflect your wisdom. You don't get smarter by aging. You get smarter by using your brain. This mentality is arrogant, but it doesn't stop there. Some adults can't even challenge their own beliefs (which is pretty important in life). They just follow the herd and keep on doing it even if it makes no sense or even if it's not even healthy. I have no clue why people tend to do this or maybe I do. Maybe we're not designed to leave our comfort zones. Maybe it's something that we've got to learn.

362. MOST ADULTS ENVY OTHER ADULTS FOR THEIR "STUFF"

Most people only care about money, fame, possessions, and things on social media (stuff like likes, followers, etc.). People think that all these things will lead to happiness, but they don't.

All of those things have one thing in common: they provide you with momentary happiness and you have to keep on buying new things or pleasing people to et the same feeling. You'll feel empty in the end. You'll be everything besides happy. It's dangerous to link your ego and happiness to stuff and still, so many people do it.

Can you guess who acts like this as well? Little kids when they've got to share their favorite toy. It's their toy and no one else's. So they have to learn to share and apparently most people unlearn this important lesson.

Let me put it this way: you're not your car. It's just a toy. You're not the likes and followers on your social media page(s).

So who are you then? Well, you are you and I suggest that you take up some self-development if you can't face yourself in the mirror.

363. MOST ADULTS CAN'T HANDLE THEIR OWN LIVES OR LIQUOR

Most adults can't handle life. They are endless victims and constantly blame other people. You don't solve a single thing by doing it, but somehow they manage to keep on doing it. These people are never happy and constantly hate on others online. It's sad, but that's what some adults do to kill time. There's a reason why I never comment or read comment sections: I don't want to argue with these people.

But it doesn't end there. Some people hate their jobs and that's why they complain so damn much. But they have a pretty simple solution to kill all the negative feelings. It's called "the weekend." So you basically get drunk twice and recover from that hangover on Sunday.

To this day, I still don't get how people can live like this. No wonder that they're going broke - they drink all their money away. The money can be invested in better things, but those people just choose to escape their own reality.

364. MOST ADULTS AVOID RESPONSIBILITIES LIKE THE PLAGUE

Part of being an adult is taking responsibility. You can't claim that you're an adult if you don't want it and most people don't want it. They want to Netflix and chill without paying a single bill. They want all the fun but to avoid all the work parts.

That's just not how it works in life. You won't get far if you don't take responsibility. You can fuck around all you want, but how can you expect to start a business, a better life or maybe a sports career if all your energy goes to partying and chasing girls? It's even worse if you keep on flirting with other girls all the time when you're in a serious relationship. I have one simple message to all the guys who avoid all their responsibilities:

"For he who makes a beast of himself gets rid of the pain of being a man."

365. JUST THINK ABOUT IT

Most adults can't handle failure nor adversity.

Ever seen how some adults handle their own failures/adversity? They shy away from their own problems and they laugh at others when they fail. This just proves that they've got a weak mindset.

But this results in some weird parenting as well. They punish kids for failing a test, so these kids link failure to bad feelings. They're conditioned to feel bad after they've failed. No wonder that most adults can't handle it. Failure can only be bad, according to adults, while it isn't if you find out why you failed.

This reminds me of the time that I dropped out of college. Most people told me that my life was officially over, whole others just ditched me because they didn't want to hang out with a loser. So many people judged me because I didn't have a clue what I want in life ,but do they know? I assume they don't, but they still judged me anyways.

It's still one of the best things that ever happened to me. You just have to change your perspective and then you can change your life. Or you can complain a whole day on Facebook and hope that people give you attention. That's a possibility as well, but it's not what grown-ups do.

366. I KNOW NOTHING ABOUT LIFE

I just shared tons of life lessons with you – 373 to be exact, because this is going to be a lesson as well.

You see, most people assume that I've got everything figured out and that my life is perfect. Well, I haven't figured life out and my life is far from perfect. I make mistakes all the time, but I take responsibility for them. I try to learn something from every mistake that I make - that's it.

It would be really arrogant for me to claim that I've got life figured out. I mean, I always feel that I know nothing when I learn something new. I'm pretty sure that you'll never stop learning in life, or at least not if you've got the right mindset.

Well, that's the final last lesson. You're almost at the end of the book!

367. LIFE LESSONS & MY GRATITUDE

I'm pretty grateful that I was able to write this book. I just gave away a lot of life lessons and I hope that they'll help you throughout your life. I'm pretty honored that you made it to the end of the book, to be honest. It's one of the biggest things that I've ever written. I'll probably never do this again because I was really sick of the writing at the end. I missed my training sessions in the gym as well.

Whatever the case, I hope you can take away something from my life, my failures and my successes.

Don't forget to leave a review on Amazon. That would be really appreciated!

Aside from that, I have a gift for you. You can download a free PDF which includes some of my training routines and favorite books. The free download also includes some tips on how to read more and never miss a workout. You can take your mind and body from Zero To Alpha with this guide, so what are you waiting for? You can download if by subscribing to my e-mail list at zerotoalpha.com.

Now it's time to hit the gym. Adios, my friends!

Yours,

Alex

www.zerotoalpha.com